TREATING PTSD IN PRESCHOOLERS

Treating PTSD
in Preschoolers
A Clinical Guide

MICHAEL S. SCHEERINGA

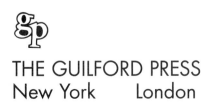

THE GUILFORD PRESS
New York   London

© 2016 The Guilford Press
A Division of Guilford Publications, Inc.
370 Seventh Avenue, Suite 1200, New York, NY 10001
www.guilford.com

Printed in the United States of America

This book is printed on acid-free paper.

Last digit is print number: 9   8   7   6   5   4   3   2   1

The author has checked with sources believed to be reliable in his efforts to provide information that is complete and generally in accord with the standards of practice that are accepted at the time of publication. However, in view of the possibility of human error or changes in behavioral, mental health, or medical sciences, neither the author, nor the editor and publisher, nor any other party who has been involved in the preparation or publication of this work warrants that the information contained herein is in every respect accurate or complete, and they are not responsible for any errors or omissions or the results obtained from the use of such information. Readers are encouraged to confirm the information contained in this book with other sources.

Library of Congress Cataloging-in-Publication Data

Scheeringa, Michael S.
    Treating PTSD in preschoolers : a clinical guide / Michael S. Scheeringa.
      pages cm
    Includes bibliographical references and index.
    ISBN 978-1-4625-2233-0 (paperback)
    1. Post-traumatic stress disorder in children—Treatment.   2. Cognitive therapy.   I. Title.
    RJ506.P55S42 2016
    618.92′8521—dc23
                                                                                2015025242

About the Author

Michael S. Scheeringa, MD, MPH, is the Venancio Antonio Wander Garcia IV, MD, Chair in Psychiatry, Vice Chair of Research, and Professor of Psychiatry and Behavioral Sciences at the Tulane University School of Medicine. His research focuses on posttraumatic stress disorder (PTSD) in youth, including preschool children, and has included large multimodal assessment studies and randomized clinical trials. He developed and tested a cognitive-behavioral therapy manual on preschool PTSD treatment, which was the basis for this book. Dr. Scheeringa also developed one of the few diagnostic assessment interviews for young children, the Diagnostic Infant and Preschool Assessment. He is currently working to support the implementation of evidence-based screening, assessment, and treatment for trauma-related problems in the child welfare system in Louisiana. Dr. Scheeringa is a Distinguished Fellow of the American Psychiatric Association and a recipient of the Irving Philips Award for Prevention from the American Academy of Child and Adolescent Psychiatry, among other honors.

Preface

The assessment and treatment of posttraumatic stress disorder (PTSD) in very young children requires special considerations due to developmental differences in cognitive, language, emotional, and behavioral capacities. For example, a 4-year-old girl who appears inexplicably terrified when her grandmother pulls out a knife in the kitchen is unable to verbalize that the knife is a trigger that reminds her of when she saw her father stab her mother to death. The 5-year-old boy who trembles with fear when it rains hard actually fears that the house will flood, as it did during the hurricane. He does not just imagine that it will flood; he *believes* that it will flood. Treatment of these children must be adapted so that they, and their caregivers, can learn new ways to process and cope with these symptoms.

Preschool PTSD Treatment (PPT) is a theory-driven, manualized protocol based on cognitive-behavioral therapy (CBT), with modifications for young children with PTSD. It was developed from years of working directly with young children and modified from lessons learned in a randomized clinical trial (Scheeringa, Weems, Cohen, Amaya-Jackson, & Guthrie, 2011). Some of these modifications involve parent–child relationship dynamics that are salient for this age group. The manual was created for use with 3- to 6-year-old children because 3 years of age is about the lower limit at which children can understand and cooperate with CBT techniques. Use with children older than 6 years, however, is quite possible with minor adaptations.

The manual is focused on a developmentally appropriate model of graduated exposure therapy, or systematic desensitization. The main process occurs in three steps. The first step is an acquisition of relaxation strategies. The second step is the development of a stimulus hierarchy list. The third step is to expose the child to fears on the stimulus hierarchy list and teach the child how to endure the anxiety by applying new relaxation skills rather than fleeing from the reminders. There are, however, many other components used before, during, and after this main therapeutic process that facilitate the success of the psychotherapy.

This manual provides detailed directions for how to conduct this form of CBT with young children. The techniques are common and fairly straightforward. The clinical skills needed to implement them with young children are often more complicated, however, so the philosophy guiding the writing of this manual was to favor clear and specific step-by-step directions. This is what I have found works best when training therapists to use this model.

I would like to particularly acknowledge Judith A. Cohen, MD, and Lisa Amaya-Jackson, MD, who were coauthors on the original version of the manual. They were very gracious in helping to launch the research study in which we first fully tested the treatment manual, and they offered the wisdom from their enormous amount of experience in working with trauma-exposed children and their families.

Carl Weems, PhD, was of singular importance during the research study. He was our expert consultant during weekly supervision meetings for the 4 years of the study. Carl helped us to hone our CBT techniques and frequently served as our voice of wisdom when faced with difficult clinical and procedural research questions.

I would also like to thank the original therapists in the research study, Alison Salloum, PhD, LCSW, and Ruth Arnberger, LCSW, and the research assistant, Tiffany Thomas. They provided many valuable suggestions and helped to develop the handouts, worksheets, and cheat sheets. Theresa Stockdreher, LCSW, the therapist for the second part of that research study, was also helpful. Also, I am very thankful to student intern Camila Woodmansee, who extracted the verbatim conversations from videotape for many of the case vignettes in the book. Many other therapists in the United States and other countries who have used the manual over the years and who are too numerous to mention have also offered feedback and suggestions, for which I am truly grateful. Thank you to artist Carol Peebles, who graciously helped us reimagine and expand the pictorial aids. My wife, Claire Peebles, PhD, a superb clinician in private practice who specializes in infant/preschool problems, was my noon and midnight triple threat of expertise, better judgment, and moral support.

A special thank-you must go to the families who allowed us to work with them and their young children. Without their participation, none of this would be possible. (Names and details of the case vignettes in this book have been changed to protect confidentiality.)

Lastly, I believe that what prevents most therapists from fully embracing evidence-based, manualized protocols, such as CBT, is that they are too hard on themselves and do not like to attempt something that they do not believe they will be successful at implementing. Rather than expect full (perfect) fidelity to the manual, I suggest that therapists commit themselves instead to the imperfect *attempt*. When it becomes apparent that children improve, it gets easier.

Contents

Contents

Purchasers of this book can download and print select materials
from *www.guilford.com/scheeringa-forms.*

PART I

Introduction and Background

CHAPTER 1

Overview of Preschool PTSD Treatment

Why Is Treatment Needed?

Natural Course

Exposure to life-threatening traumatic events is common. More than two-thirds of children experience at least one life-threatening traumatic event by age 16 years (Copeland, Keeler, Angold, & Costello, 2007). Of those, more than one-third experience more than one traumatic event. The good news is that approximately 70% of individuals appear to be resilient. The bad news is that the 30% of individuals who are susceptible to develop trauma-related symptoms often have a chronic course and need a specific type of therapy to help them recover.

Prospective longitudinal studies have demonstrated a need for treatments such as this manual by showing that posttraumatic stress disorder (PTSD) does not usually disappear with a tincture of time or even an extended period of time. Investigators have estimated the prevalence of PTSD in young children to be 10% 6 months after motor vehicle accidents (Meiser-Stedman, Smith, Glucksman, Yule, & Dalgleish, 2008) and burns (De Young, Kenardy, Cobham, & Kimble, 2012), 25% 6 months after a gas explosion in Japan (Ohmi et al., 2002), 17% 9–12 months post 9/11 (DeVoe, Bannon, & Klein, 2006), 13% on average 15 months after burn injury (Graf, Schiestl, & Landolt, 2011), and 23% 2 or more years after a variety of traumatic events (Scheeringa, Zeanah, Myers, & Putnam, 2005).

Prospective Studies in Young Children

There have been several well-done studies on the long-term trajectories of PTSD symptoms in young children. We conducted the first prospective follow-up of PTSD symptoms in a cohort of 1- to 6-year-old children (Scheeringa et al., 2005). The families were non-help-seeking and experienced a variety of types of trauma, including accidents, abuse, and witnessing domestic violence. Initially, there were 62 children in the sample with a mean of 3.6 PTSD symptoms, and 26% meet the full PTSD diagnosis. After 2 years, the 35 children retained in the sample had a mean of 2.9 symptoms, and 23% still met the full PTSD diagnosis. As there was no evidence of significance natural recovery, nearly the entire sample seemed to follow the chronic–worsening trajectory.

Meiser-Stedman et al. (2008) assessed 62 2- to 6-year-old children 2–4 weeks following motor vehicle accidents and found a 7% prevalence of PTSD. When reassessed 6 months later, the prevalence had actually increased to 10%. More encouraging, De Young et al. (2012) studied 130 1- to 6-year-old children following burn injuries and found a 25% prevalence of PTSD 1 month after the trauma, which decreased to 10% after 6 months.

The long-term trajectories of PTSD symptoms have been described mostly for adult trauma victims. Long-term follow-up studies have shown several different trajectories over time (Bonanno et al., 2012). A *moderate* group shows medium severity of PTSD symptoms and some gradual natural recovery. A *high* group shows high severity of PTSD symptoms and some gradual natural recovery. A *chronic–worsening* group shows moderate to severe symptoms and does not improve or worsens over time. Relatively few of the individuals in these groups naturally improve to achieve complete absence of symptoms. Substantial improvements are possible for some individuals, but once PTSD develops, it is a quite chronic problem.

These data make it clear that PTSD does not go away on its own and that intervention is required. When should intervention begin? Treatment is indicated if symptoms persist after 1 month. The National Institute for Clinical Excellence (2005) published an expert consensus report that stated that watchful waiting is the recommendation for mild symptoms within the first month, whereas treatment within the first month ought to be considered for severe PTSD. This recommendation was based on a very substantial body of evidence that symptoms that are present after 1 month are likely to endure, impair, and not resolve without evidence-based treatment.

Thus, contrary to a widely held belief that children simply "grow out of" PTSD (Cohen & Scheeringa, 2009), these findings indicate that a substantial proportion of trauma-exposed young children have chronic PTSD symptoms and impairment and require treatment. Furthermore, in our follow-up study, we noted that although 17 children had received community treatment, they did not improve, suggesting that community treatment as usual was ineffective and that more effective treatment was needed (Scheeringa et al., 2005). This and other considerations led us to develop the following treatment protocol.

Development of Preschool PTSD Treatment

Prior to the development of Preschool PTSD Treatment (PPT), only two randomized studies had focused on trauma-related symptoms of young children, and both were limited to those exposed to sexual abuse. Cohen and Mannarino (1996a) had randomly allocated

39 3- to 6-year-old sexually abused children to either 12 individual sessions of trauma-focused cognitive-behavioral therapy (TF-CBT) or nondirective supportive therapy. The TF-CBT group improved significantly more than the supportive therapy group on Total Behavior Problems and the Internalizing scale of the Child Behavior Checklist; a PTSD measure was not employed in this study. Deblinger, Stauffer, and Steer (2001) had randomly allocated 44 2- to 8-year-old children to either 11 sessions of group TF-CBT or group supportive educational treatment. Both groups improved on PTSD symptoms; the TF-CBT group did not show greater improvement than the supportive educational group, perhaps because the TF-CBT group members were not asked to speak about their own experiences due to their young ages.

Although both of these randomized studies with young children were encouraging, several limitations needed addressing. First, only the Deblinger et al. (2001) study used an outcome measure of PTSD and found no difference between TF-CBT and supportive groups. The evidence for reducing PTSD symptoms in young children was thus slim. Second, both studies were limited to children with sexual abuse. Thus, when the first-ever federally funded programs to train clinicians to treat children for PTSD were created, following the 2001 World Trade Center attacks and the 2004 Florida hurricanes, preschool children were left out of these large and important programs because of the perception that there were no sufficient disaster protocols for this age group (Allen, Saltzman, Brymer, Oshri, & Silverman, 2006; CATS Consortium, 2007).

An additional gap was the absence of feasibility data as to whether young children could understand and cooperate with the essential techniques of cognitive-behavioral therapy (CBT). Although the Cohen and Mannarino (1996a) and Deblinger et al. (2001) studies both used rigorous methods to ensure therapist fidelity to the treatment protocols, they did not have data on the actual feasibility of the CBT techniques for the children. In other words, the therapists appropriately followed the protocols, but there were no separate ratings on whether children appeared to understand each element of the protocol. Therapist fidelity and feasibility for children may overlap quite a bit, or they may not. Another major aim of developing PPT was to create a treatment method that was proven to have tasks that young children could really do (i.e., be developmentally feasible).

The PPT protocol was first developed based on the relevant literature about the use of CBT techniques to treat PTSD, my research findings on assessments of young children, and my clinical experience of trying to treat PTSD in young children. During the process of writing the manual, I invited Judith A. Cohen and Lisa Amaya-Jackson to assist and be coauthors. Cohen and Anthony P. Mannarino had experience in developing and testing of TF-CBT in older children. In addition, they had conducted the previously mentioned study using CBT for sexually abused children ages 3–6 years (Cohen & Mannarino, 1996a), which included, among other techniques, anxiety management training (direct discussion of trauma reminders with progressive relaxation and positive imagery), detection of distorted attributions, and time spent with the mothers over a 12-session individual therapy structure. Amaya-Jackson, with John March, had written and tested a group CBT manual for older children (March, Amaya-Jackson, Murray, & Schulte, 1998), which included, among other techniques, anxiety management training with both narrative and imaginal exposures, the stress thermometer, a stimulus hierarchy list, positive self-talk, detection of distorted thoughts, prescribed homework for *in vivo* exposure, and relapse prevention over a 14-session group therapy structure. Judy and Lisa were quite helpful in the early stages of manual development and troubleshooting with the early cases.

Based on my research (Scheeringa, Peebles, Cook, & Zeanah, 2001; Scheeringa & Zeanah, 2001; Scheeringa, Zeanah, Drell, & Larrieu, 1995) and clinical experience with this population, I modified these techniques for 3- to 6-year-old children who had experienced any type of trauma. I also included many new techniques that had not been standardized in previous trauma interventions, including psychoeducation with pictorial aids; systematic discussion of reluctance, a session for discipline plans, implementation of nearly all exercises and narrative exposures through drawings, a personalized folder to collect drawings and worksheets, systematic desensitization that started with low-anxiety-provoking exposures and worked up to high-anxiety-provoking exposures, safety plans, inclusion of parents who watched all sessions in closed-circuit TV, and planned time with parents in every session to process the protocol material.

The Evidence Base

We tested PPT in a study that included 3- to 6-year-old children who had experienced a wide range of types of traumas between 2005 and the end of 2008 (funded by the National Institute of Mental Health, R34 MH70827). Children had to be between 36 and 83 months of age at the time of the most recent trauma and at the time of enrollment. Exclusion criteria were few and included moderate mental retardation, autistic disorder, blindness, deafness, and familial inability to speak English. Also, children whose only trauma was sexual abuse were not enrolled because the two previous studies had already shown the effectiveness of CBT for treating young victims of sexual abuse (Cohen & Mannarino, 1996a; Deblinger et al., 2001).

The study was divided into two phases. In Phase 1, we treated the first six children with the manualized protocol. This phase helped us empirically discover numerous minor revisions that were helpful (e.g., the term *safe place* was not well understood, so it was changed to *happy place*). In Phase 2, we randomly assigned half of the subjects to receive treatment immediately and the other half to a 12-week wait list (WL). The duration of the 12-week WL was designed to be the same duration of time as the treatment group. Hurricane Katrina struck New Orleans soon after Phase 2 began, which interrupted the treatment of several subjects and stopped all activity for nearly 6 months as our clinic was being made habitable again. Because of this delay, we opted to allocate the next 10 subjects to immediate treatment in order to rebuild the caseloads before we resumed randomization. As a result, more children were assigned to immediate PPT treatment ($n = 51$) than to the 12-week WL period ($n = 24$). Thirty-two children completed at least one session in the PPT group, 20 completed all 12 sessions, and 11 completed the waiting period in the WL group.

The first aim of the study was to test the effectiveness of the protocol to reduce PTSD symptoms. The treatment clearly worked and the changes between these groups were highly significant (Scheeringa, Weems, et al., 2011). The PPT group had a mean of 7.9 symptoms before treatment, which decreased to a mean of 3.6 symptoms after treatment. The WL group showed no significant improvement during the waiting period (mean 7.7 PTSD symptoms prewait vs. 7.2 symptoms postwait). Also, the qualitative use of the manual was described with two case studies (Scheeringa et al., 2007).

Next, 10 of the 11 children who completed the WL period still met the study inclusion criteria, so they were treated with PPT. Six of these 10 children completed all 12 sessions, and they were then combined with the PPT group to form a single group to estimate effect sizes of the treatment. The effect size for reducing PTSD symptoms was large by conventional standards: $d = 1.01$. The number of symptoms also significantly decreased for major depressive disorder (MDD), oppositional defiant disorder (ODD), and separation anxiety disorder (SAD), but not for attention-deficit/hyperactivity disorder (ADHD). The effect sizes for MDD, SAD, and ODD were also large: $d = 0.92$, 0.72, and 0.89, respectively.

When treatment completers were followed up after 6 months ($n = 16$), the effect sizes were again moderate to large for all disorders except ADHD, indicating excellent stability of treatment gains.

The second main aim of the study was to examine the feasibility of every one of the CBT techniques we used with the young children. Forty-six children participated in at least one treatment session and were rated for feasibility on the TF-CBT techniques. Overall, children were judged to understand and complete 83.5% of the items rated (out of 1,793 possible from a total of 388 treatment sessions). An independent rater scored 30.7% of the treatment sessions from video ($n = 116$ sessions, 530 items), and this rater agreed with the therapists' ratings 96.2% of the time. The rater and therapists' interrater agreement (kappa) was substantial at 0.86. The feasibility data on specific techniques are presented later, after the techniques are described.

Since then, PPT has been used in my clinic by trainees whom I supervise, and by colleagues at Tulane and around the world. Feedback over the past 5 years has led to minor refinements. PPT has been disseminated to over 800 clinicians in 27 trainings around the world, including England and Australia, and distributed to hundreds of other clinicians via the Internet.

Who Is Appropriate for Treatment?

In our randomized trial, inclusion criteria stated that children had experienced a life-threatening traumatic event and had four or more PTSD symptoms, with at least one of them a reexperiencing symptom from DSM criterion B or an avoidance symptom from DSM-IV criterion C. A reexperiencing or avoidance symptom was required for the exposure exercises to be salient in TF-CBT. The children did not need to meet criteria for the full disorder.

The lower age limit for children was determined by the age at which they have developed autobiographical narrative memory of events and adequate verbal language. This is typically around 36 months of age (Fivush, 1993; Terr, 1988), but may be earlier in special circumstances. The upper age limit for using this protocol is more flexible. In our randomized trial, children's ages were between 3 years, 0 months, and 6 years, 11 months, at the time of the most recent trauma and at the time of enrollment, but we have used the protocol on older children outside of that trial.

A relative contraindication to attempting this treatment is children with untreated ADHD. In my experience, it is usually more helpful to treat ADHD with medication first and then start this protocol. For equivocal cases in which the ADHD is mild or it is suspected that the ADHD symptoms are PTSD-related, then it makes sense to start the protocol and see if children can cooperate.

How Is the Treatment Theorized to Work?

A review of studies on treatment for PTSD identified three factors that were involved across types of trauma treatments:

1. Emotional engagement with the trauma memory.
2. Organization and articulation of a trauma narrative.
3. Modification of basic core beliefs about the world and oneself (Zoellner, Fitzgibbons, & Foa, 2001).

PPT addresses all three of these in a CBT structure. The challenge in working with younger children is how to apply these techniques in a developmentally sensitive fashion that both the child and parent can utilize.

CBT for PTSD

CBT appears to be an effective treatment modality for PTSD because of the focus on learning theories and cognitive distortions (Foa, Keane, & Friedman, 2009; Silverman et al., 2008; Zoellner et al., 2001). Although it is not clear what causes PTSD at a neurocircuitry level, it is evident that these are new behaviors, thoughts, and feelings that were not present prior to a traumatic event and that seem to be associated with magnified and automatic cognitive processes.

Behavior therapy rests on a primary assumption that most behavior develops and is sustained through the principles of learning (Rimm & Masters, 1979). One type of learning, operant conditioning (Skinner, 1953), is particularly useful for treatment because it works by voluntary behaviors (operants) being reinforced by consequences (response). In theory, change in behavior is linked to the strength and frequency of the responses. These characteristics can be manipulated in treatment protocols.

Cognitive therapy rests on the primary assumption that individuals interpret the world through cognitive structures (schemas) that have secondary impacts on altered feelings and behaviors (Beck, 1967). Cognitions and behaviors are, of course, not independent, and theorists have sought a more realistic amalgam of the two, such as in social learning theory (Bandura, 1969).

CBT is the rational blending of both modalities, which over the past 30 years has evolved into a diverse group of interventions (Thase & Wright, 1997). The empirically driven theory and practice of CBT lend it well to systematic and structured treatment protocols.

CBT techniques can be simplified into two components: exposures (systematic desensitization and prolonged or imaginal exposure) and anxiety management training (relaxation, cognitive restructuring, and biofeedback). Empirical support exists for both categories, plus for combined treatment packages (reviewed in Rothbaum & Foa, 1996). PPT uses both techniques in a combined treatment package. Although exposures and anxiety management training are the primary techniques that are thought to decrease PTSD, there are many other aspects of PPT that go into a successful treatment package; these are described next.

Components of PPT

The main framework of the 12 sessions of PPT is presented in the following list. The sessions build on each other in the philosophy of graded exposure therapy. The skills needed before Session 2 are taught in Session 1, and so on. Regarding the exposures in Sessions 6–10, the earlier exposures are intended to be less anxiety-provoking than later exposures in order to gradually build the child's skills to cope with the most feared exposures.

- Session 1: Psychoeducation, overview.
- Session 2: Behavior management for defiance module.
- Session 3: Learn CBT tools—identify feelings.
- Session 4: Learn CBT tools—relaxation exercises.
- Session 5: Tell the story.
- Session 6: Easy narrative exposure.
- Session 7: Medium narrative exposure.
- Session 8: Medium narrative exposure.
- Session 9: Worst-moment narrative exposure.
- Session 10: Worst-moment narrative exposure.
- Session 11: Relapse prevention.
- Session 12: Review and graduation.

The titles of these sessions only describe the main focus of each session. Multiple activities take place in each session; these are described in detail in the manual in Part II. Approaches that are constants throughout the treatment and techniques that are repetitive are described next to avoid repeating them every time in Part II.

The Office

Do not keep toys and snacks in your therapy room (we use snacks during sessions but we do not store the snack supplies in the therapy room). Avoidance is part and parcel of

PTSD. Two of the PTSD symptoms include avoidance of internal and external cues that remind individuals of their traumatic events. If toys and snacks are in your room, even if they are out of sight behind cabinet doors, children will use these distractions to avoid exposures. In addition, the main job in life for young children is to play, and they will try to play if given half the chance. Perhaps most importantly, children are brought to therapy by their parents as unwilling participants, and they do not yet have the abstract understanding that therapy is a place to come and discuss emotional and behavioral problems. The way you set up the therapy room is instructional to them about how to behave. Toys and snacks in the room are a recipe for inviting unnecessary control battles.

A Straightforward Approach

Throughout every session, and especially at the very beginning, it is important to adopt a "matter-of-fact" attitude toward discussing the trauma, especially with younger children. If the child is reticent to discuss the trauma, the therapist may feel uncomfortable "pressing the issue" because the power differential of age, size, and verbal abilities are magnified relative to working with older children and adults. This need to stay focused on the issue may also feel uncomfortable to the therapist because a caregiver observes every session. If a caregiver has made clear that he or she has avoided talking about the trauma with the child, the therapist now has two patients to worry about upsetting. Humor can be used to lighten the mood. Despite these potential challenges, the success of treatment depends on the child, and perhaps the caregiver, ultimately being able to confront these memories without disabling fears and anxiety.

The Therapeutic Alliance

In my opinion, the so-called therapeutic alliance has been a bit oversold. The therapeutic alliance is of course important. In an activity that is essentially interpersonal, how could it not be important? Where it is oversold is in the sense that the alliance has to be affectively expressed or is inappropriately and artificially created. A warm and fuzzy therapeutic alliance certainly makes therapy more pleasurable. All individuals, however, are neither inherently affectively expressive nor terribly interested in interpersonal interaction (e.g., those with Asperger syndrome and its variants). Treatment can be just as successful with more affectively aloof alliances that have a solid underpinning of cooperation. When the alliance does not come so easily, the therapist must be able to adapt his or her interaction style to the temperament and personality level of each individual (not the other way around). Cooperation is the only essential aspect without which therapy cannot succeed.

Reluctance

Based on research data that showed that caregivers of children with PTSD have enormous symptomatic burdens of their own (reviewed in Scheeringa & Zeanah, 2001) and on the clinical experience that mothers are often reluctant to recollect their children's traumatic experiences, we built in motivation and compliance sections for the mothers in every session. The therapist is directed to preemptively anticipate with the mother that she will feel reluctant to come to subsequent sessions. This feeling is validated, systematically rated on a weekly basis, and addressed in more depth when needed.

Emphasis is placed on the importance of the therapist preparing parents for the possibility that they will not want to come back for subsequent sessions. This common reluctance arises for several reasons. For one, parents do not want to confront painful memories, and they do not want to put their children through painful memories. In some cases the children improve a bit and the parents use that improvement as an excuse to stop coming. Another possibility is that parents have started to dredge up traumatic memories from their own pasts. If one of these reasons stops a family from coming back for treatment, it is already too late to address it. In this protocol, the reluctance to return is anticipated and discussed in the first session and in every session thereafter. This preemptive validation of the parents' experiences has the added benefit of building their trust in the therapist's competence. It shows that the therapist has experience and even expertise in this area and knows what's coming down the road.

Parents are given directive advice to report how they ignored their reluctance and came back anyway. They are asked to report "what tricks you used to make yourself come back." Some of the "tricks" that parents have reported to us include:

- "I just come because my child needs it."
- "I took a Xanax."
- "I prayed."
- "I don't want my girl to go through what I went through" (the mother had been sexually molested as a child, as her daughter was, but the mother never received any counseling or support).
- More than one mother of boys who witnessed severe domestic violence perpetrated by their fathers said, "I don't want him to turn out like his father."

As one can see from most of these comments, the parents sacrificed their own discomfort so that their children could get help.

Candy and Snacks

The use of food is a technique to help children enjoy the otherwise unpleasant activity of talking about their traumatic experiences. Food helps break the ice and make children feel more comfortable. One piece of chewy candy (e.g., Tootsie Roll, Starburst, caramel chewies, Hershey's Kiss) is offered from a candy bowl at the beginning of each session. A snack, such as a bag of chips and a juice pouch, is offered about halfway through each session.

These treats are offered unconditionally. They are never to be used as rewards or withheld as enticements to influence participation in therapy sessions. If parents spontaneously attempt to use the food for contingent purposes, the therapists must gently intercede.

Offering snacks and drinks to parents must be a more flexible option. Routinely offering a cold drink or snack to the parent at every session is not recommended. However, if the absence of such an offering becomes an issue for needy parents, it is not expected that offering minimal snacks would pose a serious threat to the integrity of the treatment protocol.

Roadway Book

The Roadway Book is simply an inexpensive folder with three clasps to collect all of the worksheets. This book is one of several methods used to help the child develop a coherent narrative of the trauma, free of cognitive and memory distortions. Over the course of the treatment, this book, which is organized session by session in chronological order, is filled with projects and homework. Children are asked to individualize their books by decorating their covers and naming them.

The book can also serve an important function as a container of the distressing memories for the child. Although exposure is a fundamental component of CBT, overwhelming exposure is not fruitful. The book can be used symbolically to contain memories until the child is ready to deal with them. The book—and, symbolically, the memories—stay in the office. At the end of treatment, the child is given the option of taking the book home.

Discipline Plan

ODD is common in preschool children following trauma. For example, in our study of 62 trauma-exposed preschool children, ODD was present in 75% of those with PTSD and was the most common comorbid disorder (Scheeringa, Zeanah, Myers, & Putnam, 2003). In our experience, disruptive behavior is the single most common reason parents bring their young children for treatment following traumas (as opposed to PTSD symptoms). Therefore, Session 2 is devoted to this problem at the beginning and followed up in subsequent sessions. If defiance is not a problematic issue for a child, skip this session and go on to Session 3.

ODD has no single, clear etiology and is probably the common result of multiple different pathways. That is, it may occur in children with extremely difficult temperaments, regardless of how their parents manage them; it may result from extreme stress within families; or, it may result from a combination of these factors. However, in our clinical experience, defiance following trauma often has a clear thread. The parent feels guilty that the child has been through enough already and is reluctant to upset the child further by imposing discipline. Parents are quite cognizant of this dynamic and readily admit it. Fortunately, this type of defiance is usually remedied easily with parent training.

When determining target behaviors for discipline plans, it is *critical to narrow each behavior down* to a measurable, clear action that you (and more importantly, the mother) can tell, unambiguously, when it is occurring. For example, if the mother says, "He's mean," in response to being asked for a target behavior, "mean" is not a measurable or clearly identified action. Other unacceptable target behaviors include "He's aggressive," "He hits," and "He doesn't listen." Clear and measurable target behaviors include:

- "He chokes his sister."
- "He throws objects at the walls and/or people."
- "He doesn't pick up his toys after I tell him three times."

Once the target behaviors have been identified, set a goal that is easily achievable over the following week. It is much more important for children to achieve success for the first week of a discipline plan that it is to "fix" the whole problem. For example, set a goal of picking up toys after one reminder for only 2 out of the next 7 days. After this goal is met, the goal can be increased in the subsequent weeks. More often than not, given the inherently oppositional nature of many children with ODD problems, they will exceed these low goals simply because they are not supposed to exceed them.

Lastly, pick a reward through a negotiation with the children and parents. These ought to be quite small rewards, inexpensive, and therefore imminently doable. For example, children often choose to pick a movie, order pizza, or have Mom take them to the playground.

In the following weeks in which discipline plans were implemented at home, you will need to vigorously follow up on these during sessions. There are generally three possible outcomes at this point:

1. The plan was successful. —You will either need to negotiate how to modify it for the upcoming week or just leave it in place, unmodified.
2. The parent followed the plan, but the child's behavior did not improve. —You will need to decide whether to stick with the same plan another week, "ratchet it up a notch" with more potent rewards or consequences, or choose a different target behavior.
3. The parent did not follow the plan. —You will need to assertively address this issue now, rather than later. That is, put the issue of the parent's noncompliance on the table straightforwardly, as opposed to glossing over it. It is highly probable at this point that it was not an accident that the parent did not follow the plan, and it will not be followed in the future if it is not enforced. The counselor is the enforcer. You must sensitively "hold the parent's feet to the fire" and remind him or her that there are consequences—that is, the child's defiant behavior—if the parent does not follow the behavior plan.

How many weeks should discipline plans be used? As few as possible, and until the parent appears satisfied with the outcome. The typical range is one to five sessions. We do not try to keep repeating discipline for too many weeks because by Session 6 we really want the homework-related attention focused on the *in vivo* exposures.

Note on time-out: There tends to be widespread misunderstandings among both clinicians and parents about time-out. The erroneous view of time-out is that it is a therapeutic technique that has efficacy in producing long-lasting changes in behavior. Time-out may work that way in your average child who has no clinical-level disturbances, but that is not our clinical population.

The proper use of time-out with a clinical population most of the time is as a last resort measure to temporarily interrupt disobedience or to stop children from harming themselves, others, or property. *Temporarily interrupt* is the key phrase. When time-out temporarily stops a child from doing something unsuitable, by definition, it has worked. We do not use time-out to extinguish bad behavior or instill morality. If a parent says, "I tried time-out and it didn't work," then reeducate him or her on the true usefulness of time-out. We generally do not use time-outs in discipline homework, but you may still want to address it as an aside.

Grief

When a loved one has been lost in a trauma, grief can be an important issue that needs to be addressed. Grief can also be tricky for parents of young children to deal with because they are not sure whether young children should be encouraged to grieve or not. Sometimes the issue is that the parents don't want to think about the loss, and so, by proxy, they discourage the child from talking about the person and evolving through the normal grieving process.

What is the difference between normal and abnormal forms of grief? The *normal* grief response includes feelings of loneliness and preoccupation with thoughts and memories of the lost person. The responses can be grouped in the usual four categories of human responses: (1) feelings (sad and angry), (2) somatic symptoms/sensations (headaches, stomachaches, trembling, sweaty, and heart racing), (3) thoughts (missing the person and thoughts about how the person died), and (4) behaviors (crying, withdrawal, and temper tantrums).

Grief is considered *abnormal* when it has lasted abnormally long or is abnormally severe. Abnormal grief may be considered if, after 6 months, the child continues to feel persistent longing for the deceased; intense sorrow, anger, and/or self-blame; excessive avoidance of reminders of the loss; a desire to die to be with the deceased; persistently feeling alone and detached; and a loss of interest in usual activities.

Some basic tips on how to handle grief are provided in Session 2. For more extensive suggestions or guidance on complicated cases, therapists ought to consult grief-specific manuals (e.g., Salloum, 1998).

Parents Watch Sessions on TV

Sessions 3–11 begin with children, parents, and therapists checking in for 5 minutes or less. Then the parents go to a separate room and watch the therapy sessions in real time on a monitor. After the work with the children is finished, the parents come back into the room with the therapists while, ideally, the children can be in a separate room supervised by another adult. This is an unusual amount of changing rooms that requires extra effort, so why do it?

With children this young, you *must* have parents involved in some aspects of the treatment and it is ideal to have parents involved in all aspects of the treatment. So what is the best way to get parents involved? The parents need to *see* everything that you are doing with their children and learn all the same things that the children are learning. You cannot have the parents in the room with you and the children because children act and talk differently with their parents in the room. Also, you want the children involved with you during the therapy session, not the parents, so it becomes a little awkward to have the parents sitting on the side like third wheels.

We have found this method of having parents watch the sessions on TV to be helpful in multiple ways. First, young children are still developing verbal expression skills to communicate their thoughts and feelings to others. By default, you have to rely on reading their body language to know if they are anxious or avoidant. You do not know the children well enough to read their body language with that level of subtlety, but parents are experts at it. Parents know if something is wrong with their children just by a look that they probably cannot even explain. Therapists benefit by receiving this feedback from parents when the parents rejoin the therapists at the end of each session. Therapists can then use this feedback in subsequent sessions with the children.

Second, the children will need to do homework, and parents are essential to this treatment component. Parents have to understand the rationale for the homework and the steps involved because they will have to initiate the homework, transport their children to the *in vivo* exposure sties, and help guide them through the homework steps.

Third, two of the most useful ways that parents can help their children improve is by helping them avoid trauma reminders in the environment that trigger their distress, and by patiently soothing their children after they become distressed by triggers. To be able to provide these two sources of help, parents need to be better attuned to their children's internal lives. Most, if not all, parents that we have worked with have told us that they never asked their children to tell their stories of what happened to them in their traumatic events. Or, when parents thought they knew what their children remembered of witnessing traumatic events, they were then surprised to learn the details of what the children truly remember after watching the session on TV. Distressing reactions of their children to seemingly mysterious triggers were rendered no longer mysterious.

Fourth, parents learn to change their behavior by *seeing* someone else work with their children in a different way than they know how to do. It is not uncommon for therapists to think that working with parents directly to change their parenting behaviors will improve the children. However, there is very little randomized, controlled evidence that therapists can change fundamental parenting behaviors that have an impact on children's psychopathology. We shall talk later about parent–child relationship issues, but for now the main point is that the only times that I have seen parents fundamentally alter their parenting in this type of treatment is by watching live interactions of others with their children. Telling parents what to do doesn't seem to work. Explaining the importance of doing something doesn't seem to work. Parents don't know what they don't know about how to parent differently, and they can't know how to make something work with their unique children until they see someone else interact more effectively with those children.

You don't have a camera and monitor? A camcorder costs about $100 and a monitor about another $100. Including cables, discs, and accessories that may be needed, a setup costs less than $300. Therapists spend more than that on new sofas. There are other barriers? There is no way to string a cable from the camera to the monitor? There is no extra room in your clinic for the mother to watch? There is always a workaround. A hole can be drilled through a wall for a cable, or wireless signals can be used. Wireless baby monitors can be used to transmit sound and sometimes pictures. You can Skype over the Internet or use a FaceTime-enabled iPhone to connect one room to another. You can record the session on your smartphone or tablet and play back selected portions for the parents. These days there is almost no excuse to prevent showing the sessions to parents.

Scary Feelings Score (a.k.a. Stress Thermometer)

When children are called upon to do exposures during the office sessions and *in vivo* homework assignments, they need to be able to identify and communicate when their emotional distress increases from not distressed to more distressed. Conversely, after performing their relaxation exercises, they need to be able to identify and communicate when their emotional distress decreases from distressed to less distressed. Children in this age group have usually never been asked to communicate this degree of detail about their emotions, so they need to be taught the skill.

In older populations, this tool is a 10-point rating scale known as the Subjective Units of Distress Scale or more simply as a stress thermometer. We've found empirically that young children cannot grasp a 10-point scale, so we use a 3-point scale. They don't understand the word *stress*, but they usually do understand *scary feelings*. They don't understand thermometers yet.

In Session 4, therapists teach children how to rate their scary feelings, and this 3-point scale is thereafter used in a variety of in-office and homework exposures.

Relaxation Exercises

I recommend that you teach three relaxation exercises: slow breathing, muscle relaxation, and an imaginary "happy thought." All of the relaxation exercises may not work for some children, so a range of exercises is taught. It is hoped that each child finds at least one of these techniques useful.

A child may dislike all of the relaxation exercises for an idiosyncratic reason, or it may become apparent that another exercise works much better. For example, a child may get a better result from his mother rubbing his belly when he's upset. One boy created a way to interweave his fingers together that calmed him during his *in vivo* exposures. Feel free to ask caregivers for other options and substitute exercises that work. If children refuse any sort of relaxation exercise, they may still be able to cooperate with the simpler and less involved task of paying attention to the feelings in their bodies.

Start with *muscle relaxation* since this one tends to be accepted more easily by this age group than the others. See the exercise description in Therapist Form 3 in Part III for an example. This description uses counting by 2's to make it rhythmic and concrete.

We've found that it is engaging to describe this process as "making your muscles tight, *tight*" (demonstrate by squeezing your arm muscles) and then "go loose like noodles" (shake your arms around like noodles to demonstrate). You may use your own favorite method too. The point is to try to make the exercise fun and engaging.

Next, teach children about slow, controlled *breathing*. Children typically show the most resistance to this exercise. Try to make it an engaging contest about breathing in through the nose, and then out through the mouth. Show the child how to do it and use exaggerated facial expressions such as a crinkled nose and puckered mouth. Another way to make it a contest is to have them blow hard and long on something like a pinwheel or a piece of paper. Counting and tapping out beats can also make it rhythmic and easier to remember (e.g., "Breathe in, one, two, breathe out, one, two, three"). Or, suggest that the child lie down to make it more relaxing.

There is some empirical evidence (Ancoli & Kamiya, 1979; Ancoli, Kamiya, & Ekman, 1980) that recruitment of the parasympathetic branch of the autonomic nervous system, as opposed to the sympathetic branch, for breathing has a more calming effect (although that evidence does not come from work with trauma-exposed youth). The parasympathetic branch may be recruited by using the diaphragm muscle to breathe rather than the muscles in the chest wall. Diaphragmatic breathing expands the stomach during inhalation. Children can feel this expansion by simply placing their hands on their stomachs and feeling them rise and fall with each breath. However, based on experience, diaphragmatic breathing is difficult to learn and has not been shown to have a superior effect. Still, it may be worthwhile to teach.

Next, explain *happy-place imagery*. Children can learn to self-soothe when they get too scared by replacing scary feelings with an image/picture of something that makes them happy. You could call it "happy place" or "happy thought," or you may need a different term that they understand better (we initially tried "safe place," but children did not feel that *safe* was better than *happy*). A happy thought can be about some event that was fun, such as a party; or someplace calm, like the beach; or someplace familiar, like their mother's lap; or someplace private, such as a favorite window seat in their home. Young children do not associate thoughts of being alone as happy thoughts because they are so rarely alone at this age, and many are still concerned, to some degree, by separations. Younger children's happy thoughts will tend to focus on exciting events with other people. When one young girl picked the toy aisle at Walmart as her happy place, her mother protested to the therapist that the girl was not taking this seriously and was trying to get some toys out of this somehow. The therapist reassured the mother that her daughter's choice was developmentally appropriate.

If children have difficulty imagining a scene with their eyes closed, it might help to practice this skill with them. Tell them to look at a poster on your wall and then close their eyes but keep that picture of the poster in their head. With their eyes closed, quiz them about what's on the poster. Do this a few times until they can tell you what's on the poster with their eyes still closed.

These exercises are initially introduced to children as "relaxation exercises" because *relax* is a term that children this age can understand fairly easily. A proviso, however, is that *relaxation* may not be a realistic concept for this population. Children with PTSD feel genuine fear from their triggered reminders of the traumatic events they experienced. Although the exposure exercises are not intended to trigger that degree of distress, the exposures nonetheless trigger substantial amounts of anxiety. Children can decrease the amount of anxiety they feel with these exercises, but they *never* achieve a state of true relaxation. If you find that certain children resist using the exercises, consider reframing them as "body control" or "body power" activities and avoid using the term *relax*.

Stimulus Hierarchy

The "stimulus hierarchy" is simply a list of reminders/triggers arranged from the least scary to the most frightening. This list will be used to select items for office exposures and for *in vivo* homework exposures. Examples of items that work well in stimulus hierarchies can be gleaned from the real examples of office and homework exposures in the next section on exposures.

You need to take notes during Session 4 when caregivers give you their version of the trauma (see the section on getting the "bird's-eye view" in Session 4, p. 83) and during Session 5 when children tell their version of the story for the first time. The items for the stimulus hierarchy will be pulled from your notes.

What if children had more than one traumatic event in their lives? Can you mix and match events on the stimulus hierarchy? The stimulus hierarchy can include reminders from more than one event. Discuss with the children (and/or the caregivers) which single event was the scariest or most memorable, and start with that one. If children spontaneously start talking about additional events, allow them to do this freely. A rule of thumb that has worked for us is that if parents are organized enough to return phone calls and show up for appointments, they can handle multiple *in vivo* homework assignments for two different types of traumas. If parents are not able to return phone calls and show up for appointments, you ought to stick to working on one type of traumatic event at a time; if you get through the protocol for one traumatic event, the number of sessions can always be extended to work on a second traumatic event.

A common question is whether the items on the stimulus hierarchy should reflect the events that happened in the past or situations in the present that trigger reminders of the past. That is a difficult question to answer in the abstract. The answer depends on the specific details of each situation. In general, we have found from experience that the hierarchy works best as a tool in psychotherapy if it includes events from the past, not memories of the past or reminders of the past in the present day. Let's take the example of a child who had been in a motor vehicle accident. An exposure to that event from the past would be an exposure to the actual place where the accident occurred. An exposure to a reminder in the present would be an exposure to riding in a car that is not the car in which the actual accident occurred. Both types of exposures can be effective, but the exposure to the event from the past tends to have more salience.

Also keep in mind which types of situations can be turned into homework exposures and which types might be physically impossible. For example, if an event occurred in a different state, it may be impossible to do an *in vivo* exposure around many aspects of that event.

For a vertical stimulus hierarchy, list moments from the least scary to the scariest. This sheet is put in the Roadway Book and used in later sessions. It is quite important that the reminders are listed in the correct order so that sessions are focused efficiently on the most anxiety-provoking situations.

What if the child rates all reminders the same? We've found that some children rate everything as the scariest. One possible solution is to ask the caregiver to decide which are really the least and the most distressing. Another solution is to create a horizontal hierarchy instead of a vertical one.

Regardless of whether a vertical or horizontal hierarchy is created, the determination that you are on the right track is always a bit of trial and error. Using all available information from the caregivers and children, make your best guess about which events on the hierarchy to focus and then reevaluate after each session to determine if these are provoking sufficient anxiety to be effective. In a case that we published (Scheeringa et al., 2007), we initially thought that a boy's worst moment had been separation from his mother when he was put in a boat with his grandparents to leave their flooded house during the Hurricane Katrina disaster. We had chosen the separation event as a best guess based on information provided mainly by his mother. As the therapy proceeded, however, the boy spontaneously turned the lights off in the therapy room a couple of times, which cued the therapist to ask if he was afraid of the dark, to which he agreed. This also led his mother to reconsider the past events and realize that it had been extremely frightening when the family had lived in their attic in the dark for 2 days and nights to escape the floodwater. They shifted the experience of being in the attic to the top of his stimulus hierarchy, and his symptoms subsequently improved dramatically.

Exposures/Narratives/Drawings

Nearly all of the tasks for children to complete in the PPT manual involve drawing. Drawing is a common technique used to assist younger children with recall of past memories, to help express internalized thoughts and feelings (Gross & Hayne, 1998), and in particular to facilitate the expression of painful traumatic memories (Malchiodi, 1997; Steele, 2012).

Drawing is also a highly developmentally appropriate way to interact with young children. Having something on the table that is between the children and therapists, which gives the children something to focus on, is a great facilitator for communication. It is developmentally inappropriate to expect young children to sit in a chair and make eye contact with an adult and hold a back-and-forth conversation. Young children do not yet have the capacities or practice to do that. The easiest communications will always occur when there is something between the therapists and children such as drawings or worksheets.

Easy items that the child can already tolerate fairly well are picked first in Session 6. You will work together over Sessions 6–10, moving up the list toward the "worst moment." Do not let overly eager children pick their worst moment for their first exposure practice because they do not have the capacity yet to understand for what they are volunteering. There will be plenty of repetition in later sessions to get to the worst moment. Conversely, you may need to encourage anxious children to move more quickly up the list.

Producing the ideas for the children's exposures often requires creativity. To help with that, the drawing/narrative exposures conducted in the office and the homework exposures that we've done with actual patients are listed for various types of traumatic events in the section titled "Tips on Creating Drawings/Narratives and Homework for Different Types of Traumatic Events."

When starting the first exposure, *explain* that children are going to start making their scary feelings (PTSD) go away. They will need to pick an easy item from their list, draw it, then imagine it, and tolerate the anxiety until their fear goes down. For this easy task, this may not take long.

Ask the child to *draw* a picture of this item. Give the child the worksheet for the Roadway Book with empty space for drawing (Child Worksheet 6.1). This is titled the Not-Too-Scary Reminder. The purpose is for the child to stay mentally in the situation until he or she is not scared at all and may even get bored. Overall, this activity ought to last several minutes, or the amount of time it takes to draw the picture. The child can use the relaxation exercise to help him or her stay with the scene until the scary feelings go away. This sounds simple, but it can be a rather long affair for children who have difficulty and need guidance on what and how to draw. For children who simply can't or won't do the drawing, you can do the drawing and narrate out loud as you go. Other children may take a long time because they want to spend a lot of time on the drawing. Have patience.

Ask for the *scary feelings score* at the beginning for a baseline rating and then every 3–5 minutes thereafter. "How scared are you now—none, a little, or a lot?" Keep a copy of the scary feelings score in view on the table for the child to reference. We've found that we need to be a bit leading with young children because they do not have fully developed skills yet for the metacognitive task of self-monitoring their internal states and then reporting these states to another person. They need some scaffolding to understand this exercise. It is useful to remember that in the early sessions you are probably *educating* the child on how to do this exercise as much as anything. We approach it in a two- or three-step ritual:

1. Before asking the child for his or her rating, ask, "Did that make you feel more nervous? Did your scary feeling score go up?"
2. Then ask the child to point on the rating sheet to the face that matches how he or she feels. The child can also hold up the number of fingers: one, two, or three.
3. If the child has finished the drawing and the score is still "a lot scared," or the child seems particularly anxious before the drawing is finished, say, "Now, we're going to do one of our tools to make the scary feelings go away."

Do the relaxation exercises, even if the child claims not to be anxious, for two reasons: (1) practice, and (2) more than likely, he or she was anxious but wouldn't admit it.

Record the child's scores on the Scary Feelings Scores form (Therapist Form 1: Reluctance Checklist). These systematic data will help you judge whether the exposure task is having its intended purpose (to create some anxiety that rises and then falls).

Watch out for some children, particularly boys, who don't want to admit to being scared. If you suspect this is happening, change *your* wording from "How scared are you?" to "How *hard* was that—none, a little, or a lot?" Some children feel relatively more anger than fear from these exposures. If you only use the words *scared, nervous,* or *anxious* with them, the task may not have the needed salience, and it will look like it is not working for them. If this appears to be the case, consider using an emotion word that more accurately reflects the feelings stirred up by the reminders. If it's not fear or nervousness, it is usually anger, but it could be sadness or some other negative emotion. Older children can adapt on their own if you are using the wrong emotion words, but preschool children tend to follow your directions more literally.

After completing this drawing, ask children to close their eyes and think about it for 30 seconds for an *imaginal exposure*. This may seem redundant, and it is. It is meant to create more exposures while changing things up a bit. In addition, imaginal exposures may be easier or more productive for some children.

Tips on Creating Drawings/Narratives and Homework for Different Types of Traumatic Events

The following descriptions of cases, drawings, and homework assignments are derived from work with actual patients. Identifying details have been changed in all examples to protect the personal information of the individuals.

Sexual Abuse

This 3-year-old girl suffered sexual abuse from an adult male who was not a family member at a location outside of the home.

Session	Drawing/narrative	Homework
6	Sitting in the room in the house where the abuse occurred, just before it happened.	Mom and child drive past the house where it happened but do not stop.
7	Driving in Mom's car to the house where it happened.	Mom and child drive to the house where it happened and stop to sit in the car outside.
8	Picture of the perpetrator.	Sit in car outside the house where it happened. Make it more intense by sitting there longer.
9	Room where abuse occurred.	Drive to house where abuse occurred and get out of car briefly.
10	Child lying down, perpetrator standing next to her.	Get out of car at house again. Do it for a little longer than last time.
11	Near future: Next week, going to a new house. Distant future: Next month, going to a new house.	Get out of car at house again. Do it for a little longer than last time.

Domestic Violence

This child witnessed many instances of domestic violence that culminated in his mother being shot by his father when he was 5 years old. The shooting incident was immediately preceded by an argument between the mother and father in their car, in which their car hit a telephone pole in front of their house (the child was not in the car). The mother then ran into the house where she was shot in front of the children. The children fled the house through the front yard. These types of details are important for helping to provide structure for the children, walk them through the events, and heighten the intensity of the exposures. His mother survived the shooting, and she brought him for treatment when he was 6 years old.

Session	Drawing/narrative	Homework
6	Outside of the house, car, telephone pole.	Drive to the old house and sit in the car.
7	Children running from the house into the front yard.	Drive to old house. Increase intensity by having the mother talk to the child about events, and having the child touch the telephone pole.
8	Drew himself after the shooting feeling sad about not being able to see his mom. Second drawing on what he imagined his mom looked like when she was shot.	At the old house, get out of the car, walk onto the driveway.
9	Actual scene of the shooting with Mom, Dad, and siblings.	Increase the anxiety by looking through house windows (nobody lives in the old house).
10	Add detail to the scene of the shooting with furniture and police.	Unable to look in windows of old house; somebody moved into the house.
11	Near future: Next week, Mom arguing with another adult. Distant future: Next year, neighbor woman fighting with her husband.	Drive to old house, sit in car. Increased intensity by talking about the incident for about 1–2 minutes.

Domestic Violence and Motor Vehicle Accident

This child witnessed domestic violence (DV) between his mother and father from 1 to 3 years of age and was in a motor vehicle accident (MVA) with his mother at 3 years of age. At 4 years of age, he was in the custody of his maternal grandmother, who participated in the therapy with him.

Session	Drawing/narrative	Homework
6	MVA: Mom and himself in car.	MVA: Listen to sirens. This happened naturalistically by their home.
7	DV: Mom and dad fighting.	DV: Look at an old photo of mother's bruises after a fight.
8	DV: Mom's bruised face after the fight.	DV: Look at an old photo of mother's face after a fight.
9	MVA: A truck hitting their car.	MVA: Find a truck that looks similar to the one in the MVA. Either drive up to it or walk up to it for 1–2 minutes.
10	MVA: Driving with car spinning.	DV: Stand in the bedroom where parents fought and think about the fight.
11	Near future: Next week, Mom getting a phone call from Dad and he's angry. Distant future: Next year, driving in the car and it starts swerving.	DV: Create a pretend phone call between grandmother and mother that seems stressful.

Motor Vehicle Accident

This child was a passenger in his mom's car when the car stalled at a stoplight and was rear-ended by a white pickup truck. He was 4 years old at the time of the accident and the treatment.

Session	Drawing/narrative	Homework
6	White pickup truck.	Find a white pickup truck and stand near it for 1–2 minutes.
7	White pickup truck at a stoplight.	Get closer to a white pickup truck and touch it.
8	Mom's car and white pickup truck.	Because last homework was very intense, repeat it: Touch a white pickup truck again.
9	Mom's car, white pickup truck, and the stoplight.	Drive through the stoplight where the accident happened.
10	Mom's car, white pickup truck, and the stoplight.	Drive through the stoplight where the accident happened. By chance, they also witnessed another accident at a stop sign.
11	Near future: Next week, seeing a white truck at a stoplight. Distant future: Next month, Mom's car stalling at a stop sign.	Drive through the stoplight again. The parent was too anxious to do the homework, so the grandparents drove for the homework.

MVA *Plus Medical Treatments*

This boy was a passenger in his mom's car that flipped on an interstate highway. He suffered a severe injury to an extremity that required repeated trips to the doctor for painful and scary medical treatments. He was 6 years old at the time of the accident and the treatment.

Session	Drawing/narrative	Homework
6	The restaurant that he and his mom stopped at before the accident.	Drive to a restaurant that resembles the real one and visualize being at the restaurant before the accident.
7	Mom's car on the highway.	Drive through the scene of accident.
8	Their car plus several other cars on the highway.	Drive by the actual restaurant at which they stopped, and then drive by the scene of accident. Look at the tire skid marks on the pavement.
9	Multiple scenes: Receiving emergency medical treatment at the scene, the ambulance, getting stuck by a needle in the emergency room, and wearing the neck brace.	Use an actual doctor visit that was planned the next week.
10	Lying in the car right after the accident.	Use actual doctor visit that was planned the next week.
11	Near future: Next week, going to the doctor. Distant future: As a teenager, riding in a car that swerves on the highway.	Go to actual doctor's office.

MVA *Pedestrian*

This child was 3 years old when he was playing with a football in his front yard and was struck by a car when he chased the ball into the street. The car knocked the child into a row of bushes. He now refuses to play in his yard. Treatment started when he was 4 years old.

Session	Drawing/narrative	Homework
6	Playing football in the front yard.	Go into the front yard.
7	Playing football in the front yard with more detail.	Walk around the front yard with parent and toss the football several times.

8	The front yard, the street, and the row of bushes.	Play football in the front yard; have Mom talk to child about the bushes.
9	Added the car to the scene and how he got hit.	Stand in the bushes where he was found.
10	Car hitting him and knocking him into the bushes.	Go to the bushes, play football in the front yard, talk about the accident.
11	Near future: Standing close to the curb and car whizzes past. Distant future: As a teenager, crossing a busy street.	Go to the bushes, play football in the front yard, talk about the accident.

Crime Scene Where Father Was Murdered

When this child was 5 years old, her father was murdered on a city street. The mother and child drove to the crime scene late that night. The mother got out of the car to identify her husband's body, but the children stayed in the car with another relative. The child saw police, flashing lights, yellow crime scene tape, and a crowd. It's not clear if she actually saw any part of the father's body on the ground. The child also saw a newspaper story photo of the crime scene the next day. It was difficult to tell if the crime scene had scared the child. The child was nervous about visiting the father's grave for unclear reasons (perhaps because she never saw his body, or perhaps because her mom was nervous), so this was incorporated into the homework. Treatment started when the child was 6 years old.

Session	Drawing/narrative	Homework
6	Driving over the Mississippi River bridge to the crime scene.	Redrive part of the route to get to the crime scene. Drive over the bridge, but don't go to crime scene yet.
7	Mom getting out of the car at the crime scene and blood on the street at the scene.	Drive on street near the scene and talk about what happened.
8	Father's funeral.	Visit father's grave.
9	Sitting in the car in front of the police station.	Park in front of police station. Have them talk about the incident to heighten the focus.
10	Father's funeral; crime scene again.	Visit father's grave.
11	Near future: Next week, seeing a crime scene. Distant future: As a teenager, attending a funeral.	Drive as close as possible to the old crime scene and get out of car, talk about what happened.

Frightening Story Overheard and Anxiety Sensitivity (Afraid of Becoming Afraid)

This 5-year-old boy was going to the bathroom in a stall at his school when three older boys came into the dark, creepy restroom and did not notice that he was in there. They dared each other to recite a phrase that would make a ghost come out of the hissing air vent in the wall and would capture children. One of the boys recited the phrase and then they ran out of the restroom. The child was terrified because he thought the events were really happening and he feared for his life. He became fearful of all public bathrooms and some features of that bathroom in particular. This child also had *anxiety sensitivity*, which means that he was afraid of becoming afraid. This added sensitivity probably explained why this child was vulnerable to developing symptoms from this type of incident in the first place. It was decided to structure some of the exposures around the boy's own anxiety about becoming afraid rather than focusing on reminders of the event.

Session	Drawing/narrative	Homework
6	Three boys in the bathroom.	Stand in his bathroom at home with Mom visible outside in the hallway.
7	The boy who told the story.	Stand in home bathroom, with Mom out of sight; turn out some of the lights.
8	The creepy air vent and lights in the bathroom.	Go stand in a public restroom for 1–2 minutes.
9	The three boys and the one telling the story. Include his anxiety about becoming nervous.	Use a public restroom. Include his anxiety about becoming nervous.
10	Boys in bathroom with more details.	Return to the school bathroom with Mom.
11	Near future: Next week, watching something scary on TV. Distant future: As a 20-year-old, listening to someone tell a ghost story.	Return to the school bathroom with Mom; include his anxiety about becoming nervous.

Hostage

This child was 3 years old when a criminal running from the police held her day care hostage. The staff was threatened with a gun. A glass window shattered when the criminal shot at the police through it. There was a thunderstorm that day, and she associated thunderstorms with the event.

Session	Drawing/narrative	Homework
6	She and her sibling at the day care.	Drive past the day care, talk about the glass, and talk about getting out of the day care safely.
7	The shattered window.	Stop at the day care for 1–2 minutes and talk about what happened.
8	She, her sibling, and the bad man at the day care.	Go to the day care, get out of the car, and stand on the sidewalk.
9	The bad man threatening to shoot staff.	The assigned homework was to visit the day care again, but a thunderstorm happened by chance that week which served as a sufficient homework exposure.
10	Several of the children cried, and they were all scared.	Mom found a building with a broken window like the one at the day care. They drove to it and remembered the day care for 1–2 minutes.
11	Near future: Next week, thunderstorm when she's at kindergarten. Distant future: Next year, when she's at school and hears police sirens.	Drive to old day care and walk inside.

Rode Out Hurricane; Trapped in Floodwater; Airlifted from Roof of School Shelter by Helicopter; Overwhelmed in Evacuation Crowd Waiting for Buses; Scared in Mass Evacuation Shelter

This 5-year-old child experienced numerous scary events during the weeklong Hurricane Katrina event. She saw snakes and dead animals in the floodwater. This example illustrates how complex disasters can be.

Session	Drawing/narrative	Homework
6	Mass evacuation shelter.	View picture of mass shelter.
7	School shelter.	Drive to the school shelter.
8	Crowd waiting for the buses.	Drive to the school shelter again.
9	First boat they took through the floodwater.	Drive by the site where they waited for the buses.
10	Helicopter ride.	The assigned homework was to go see a boat, but a thunderstorm happened by chance which provided a sufficient homework exposure.
11	Near future: Next week, rain. Distant future: As a 16-year-old, hurricane.	Go see the boat at a neighboring house that was used to rescue them.

Disaster: Children Who Had Not Been in Harm's Way

One of the important findings of our work after Hurricane Katrina was that young children whose families had evacuated prior to the storm and had never been in harm's way developed PTSD after they returned and witnessed their devastated homes (Scheeringa & Zeanah, 2008). The appearance of PTSD symptoms in children who had escaped the hurricane happened so many times that it did not appear to be a fluke of a few children. The onset of their symptoms was carefully tracked to the day they returned and stood on the curb outside their old homes or stepped inside their gutted homes and witnessed the loss of everything they had known there.

The mechanism of how PTSD developed in these cases is interesting. The development of PTSD requires at least a moment of panic or terror when one fears for one's life or personal safety. All of these children had already seen images of the disaster on television and doubtless knew that they were going to see their homes in some state of ruin. We cannot be sure what these children thought during these moments that may have led to the development of PTSD. One speculation is that when children saw their devastated homes in person, they finally realized that if their parents had not evacuated them, they would have been in danger; they could have been covered in mud and mold, just like their stuffed animals and toys lying all over the ground. Another speculation is that in witnessing the immensity of the destruction to their personal possessions firsthand, they suddenly believed that they were no longer safe. The next rainstorm could be another Katrina. Every rainstorm could be a Katrina.

Evacuated and Then Returned to See Destroyed Home

This child was evacuated with his family before Hurricane Katrina. Their home was flooded by over 4 feet of water and completely destroyed with mud on the floor, mold on everything, and broken furniture. He was 6 years old at the time of the flood and the treatment.

Session	Drawing/narrative	Homework
6	Stuffed animal covered with mold.	Look through the window of a house that was damaged by Katrina.
7	Child's toys that were destroyed by the flood.	Go to a store and look at toys similar to those that he had lost in the storm.
8	Decorations on wall inside house that were destroyed.	Walk through the house that has been cleaned and gutted to the studs.
9	Child's broken and moldy bed.	Look at pictures of his house when it was damaged.
10	Living room with mold and furniture tossed around and broken.	Because home exposures seemed to have worked but then lost their intensity, exposure target switched to water. Drive to the lake, look at the water, and talk about the hurricane.

| 11 | Near future: Next week, rainstorm. Distant future: As a teenager, hurricane evacuation. | Go to the lakefront where homes were destroyed and go to the water's edge. |

What If a Child Dissociates in Session?

Among the dozens of children whom we have treated with this protocol, we have seen a child appear to dissociate during a session only once. This child froze in place and stared at the wall for approximately 10 seconds during an in-office exposure. He had been doing this at home for months, so this was not a new symptom. As treatment progressed, these freezing spells gradually disappeared.

There is little written about what works best with young children who dissociate. My advice is to gently talk to the child to try to orient him or her back to the present. The sound of your voice should make the child realize that he or she is in an office with another person, and not actually reliving the traumatic event. You might say things such as, "Andrew, why don't you do your breathing?" and "Alice, are you thinking about what happened?"

When the child has stopped the freezing spell, ask what he or she was thinking about to see if the child can verbalize what just happened. Also, provide praise for using newly acquired skills to cope with it by calming him- or herself. That ought to be the last in-office exposure for the session.

When the child returns for the next session, be sure to check in with the caregiver to see if the freezing spells had increased, decreased, or did not change over the week. If the spells increased, you probably want to slow down the intensity of the in-office exposures and build in more feelings of safety in the session. Otherwise, stick to the protocol and plow ahead.

What If a Child Appears to Fabricate or Have Distorted Memories?

Shawna was a 5-year-old girl who had lived through a series of life-threatening experiences in New Orleans during the Hurricane Katrina disaster. She and her mother had nearly drowned as their house was flooded on the first day of the disaster, then they were shuttled to dry ground on two different boats through the floodwaters during which she saw dead bodies and people screaming for help. They sheltered in a school, from which they were eventually air-lifted from the roof by a rope-seat into a helicopter, only to be deposited amidst a frightening crowd amassed along a highway to wait for evacuation buses. During therapy sessions Shawna claimed that she saw her grandmother dead and floating in the water, and that an alligator grabbed the body. Her mother confirmed that the grandmother had drowned in the flood but in a completely different neighborhood. How vigorously should one address these false recollections?

The image of her grandmother's body could certainly qualify as a traumatic image, and one that could create disturbing symptoms, one of which appeared to be a serious distortion of reality. As noted earlier, the review by Zoellner et al. (2001) identified three factors that were involved across successful treatments of PTSD; one of them was the organization and articulation of a trauma narrative. One might infer from this review that this distortion in Shawna's narrative ought to be countered and corrected. There are, however, few empirical data available to make generalizations about distorted memories of young children. It was possible that Shawna's image of her grandmother was more comforting to her than the alternative of not knowing what had happened to her. Imagining that she saw her body at least allowed a lesser degree of uncertainty.

With Shawna we adopted a strategy of gently questioning her for details but not implying that her memory was incorrect. We explored rather than argued. By Session 10, Shawna's exposure narrative had become noticeably more orderly and accurate. Her mother, after watching on TV, remarked, "She's thinking today." Her symptoms, not coincidentally, had also markedly improved. It was as if, according to Zoellner et al. (2001), the trauma narrative had become more organized in the child's mind.

Homework

Homework involves *in vivo* exposure, which is probably the most effective aspect of the whole therapy because exposure to anxiety-provoking situations in real life tends to give children the best experience of managing their fears. *In vivo* exposures work just like in-office exposures, except the anxiety-provoking stimuli are out in the community. Children are expected to expose themselves to the stimuli, think about the traumatic events, rate the severity of their feelings, and then use their relaxation exercises to calm down. The whole process does not need to take more than a minute but often lasts several minutes.

Keep an eye out for the subset of children who have *anxiety sensitivity* (Weems, Costa, & Watts, 2007). That is, they get anxious about becoming anxious. They will get so worked up about the prospect of doing any exposures that might make them anxious that they can't ever get to the point of actually doing the exposures. If you suspect that this sensitivity is present, investigate systematically, and as soon as possible, by interviewing the mother to confirm or disconfirm it from past history. If anxiety sensitivity appears to interfere, then candidly ask the child about this experience, and this can then become the actual early target for homework.

Explicitly limit caregivers to do homework only one time in the next week. There is a subset of caregivers who will either misunderstand this homework or deliberately do it differently no matter how persuasively you explain it. The worst-case scenario is a caregiver who jumps the gun and decides to start breaking his or her child of a phobia. For example, one caregiver decided to try to cure her child of being afraid of the dark immediately by placing her child in a dark room and telling the child to use the exercises daily. This tactic was inappropriate, too fast, too scary, and had the potential to sabotage the rest of treatment. Another caution is that if caregivers conduct the exercises incorrectly for some reason, you don't want them doing that daily. There is absolutely no reason to assign homework more than once per week.

Whether the homework is accomplished or not depends largely on the caregivers when working with children in this age group. We've had excellent success at getting homework completed; however, there is a subset of caregivers who either forget or avoid it. The best strategy for coaxing caregivers to be more cooperative with homework has been to troubleshoot and revise assignments coupled with persistent reminders that the homework is important if their children are to get better. Some caregivers seem to respond better if the homework is presented more formally as a "contract" or "deal."

Child Cooperation

I tell therapists that 50% of the battle is to get cooperation from the children. That is true for psychotherapy for all ages because psychotherapy is a voluntary activity, but it has unique challenges with very young children.

Many young children are relatively unfocused, uncooperative, and energetic in the office for the first two to three sessions. They often settle down quickly as they learn the routine. They also settle down in Session 3 and beyond because that is when the caregivers start going into the next room and the children are alone with the therapists. In most cases, no special plan is needed to manage this behavior if it can be waited out. Have patience.

What if you've got an oppositional child who won't cooperate with the exercise? Try the following tricks.

Tell, Don't Ask

Don't *ask* the child to do the exercise. *Tell* the child (politely). The "tell, don't ask" strategy is actually appropriate for all children. And think of your alternative—what if you ask and the child says, "No"? What would be your move after that?

> Ashton was a 4-year-old who had been kicked and thrown against walls by a day care assistant on several occasions when he disobeyed her and had tantrums. During Sessions 3, 4, and 5, the therapist had tried asking him questions to do a variety of tasks.
>
> The therapist asked, "Ashton, can you think of a happy place?"
>
> "No."
>
> After several minutes of negotiation, she obtained some semi-agreement about a potential happy place. "Can you draw you in your happy place?"
>
> "No."
>
> By Session 6, the therapist had learned to "tell, don't ask" to get better cooperation. When it came time for him to draw his exposure, she stated, "Ashton, it's time for you to draw the front of your old school."
>
> Not being quite so easy to say no to that, he sat and looked at her.
>
> "Here's brown. I think that's a good color. Show me how you make a building."
>
> He picked up the brown marker and started drawing a square building.

The Time Limit

This method can work for highly anxious children who believe that when you tell them to do exposures, they will be stuck doing exposures for long stretches of time. This kind of thinking is a form of catastrophizing. Before telling them to start an exposure, strike a deal with them that they have to do the exposure for only, say, 2 minutes. Usually, they do the exposure for 2 minutes, realize that they are not overwhelmed, and are then willing to keep going. Also, young children do not have the ability to tell time on a wall clock and cannot tell when 2 minutes have passed. Do not, however, renege on the deal. If children ask you if 2 minutes have passed, you must honor the deal and preserve their trust for the next session.

The exposure component can also be turned into a sort of fun and cooperative task. Use a clock with a second hand and teach them how to tell when a minute has passed. They can do the exposure while they watch the second hand spin around, and they can be in charge of telling you when the time is up.

The Tom Sawyer Method

This method is well suited for children who are very controlling. In Mark Twain's book *Tom Sawyer*, Tom faced "deep melancholy" at the prospect of having to whitewash the picket fence. To avoid this fate, he pretended to enjoy the work in order to trick his friends to take over the job from him. Therapists can employ this tactic by acting indifferent about children's participation. Make no eye contact, start doing the drawing exposure alone, and act like you're having fun. Provide a running commentary of what you're doing. The idea is that if you act like you don't want the child to cooperate, the controlling nature of the child will do the opposite of what you appear to want.

> Four-year-old Lucy had suffered physical abuse and also witnessed her mother's boyfriend, Bobby, beating her mother and then getting arrested by the police. She became emotionally dysregulated at the mention of doing exposures in the office. She would become loud and talkative and wander around the room. The therapist could not make her physically come to the table to work on drawing the exposure. Instead, the therapist started doing the exposure drawing herself and talked out loud about what she was drawing.
>
> "Here is the police car. Here is the policeman coming to arrest Bobby," the therapist said as she drew the car and the policeman. The girl wandered over to peer at the drawing, which now appeared to be the most fun thing in the room.
>
> The girl said, "It's not a policeman. It's a policewoman."
>
> "Oh. Um, well, let's see then, she needs. . . ."
>
> "She needs a button on her shirt," said the girl, who had now sat down on the chair next to the therapist and watched intently what was being drawn.
>
> At this point, even though the therapist was doing the drawing, the child was clearly participating in an exposure.

Betcha Can't

This method is well suited for competitive children. When children refuse to cooperate and act as if they already know this and already know that and don't need to do the silly things you're telling them do, then use their competitive nature to your advantage. Turn the task into a competition. As with the Tom Sawyer tactic, it helps to act indifferent about his or her participation and make little eye contact. Oppositional children are typically competitive.

Bryce was a 5-year-old boy who had witnessed many episodes of domestic violence between his mother and father. The worst episode occurred when his father punched his mother in the face and she fell unconscious on the floor. She had a grotesque black eye for days afterward. He refused to participate in either the drawing exposure or relaxation exercises for Sessions 6 and 7, although he admitted that talking about it made him upset. For Session 8 the therapist tried the "betcha can't" tactic.

"Today, we need to draw your mom's face after the fight with dad. I don't think you'll like this." Bryce was sitting on the sofa as usual, instead of seated at the table. Whereas Bryce would have typically argued with the therapist over the activity, this time he was caught off guard and sat silently looking at her. You could almost see the wheels turning his head, trying to figure out this new challenge.

As the therapist began to draw, paying little attention to Bryce, she said, "I want the orange pencil. Orange is my favorite color. You probably don't have a favorite color."

"My favorite color is blue," Bryce said reflexively with his usual argumentative voice. The trick had worked. He was providing the information the therapist wanted even though he didn't want to provide it. The therapist just needed to keep the format intact.

"Mmmm," she replied. She worked on drawing Bryce's mother's face for 15 seconds, and then said in a low, casual voice, "Wow, this is harder than I thought. Kinda good I didn't ask you to do this one."

With that, Bryce's competitive nature simply could not resist walking over to look at this apparently impossible drawing. "That's not how she looked," he argued.

"Well, sure. Here's the black eye," she shot back.

"It's too small," he said with as much sneering tone as a 5-year-old can muster.

"There," she said, enlarging the black eye slightly. "But the hair. Hair is hard. I better do the hair too."

At this point, Bryce could resist showing her up no longer. "Let me do it," he said with exasperation. "You don't know what her hair looks like."

This strategy worked well enough so that Bryce cooperated for a couple of minutes on the drawing. One would prefer that the exposure be longer than a couple of minutes, but a couple of minutes were better than nothing. The same strategy was used to get Bryce to use the relaxation exercises.

Less Is More

This strategy is useful for nearly all types of uncooperative children, but it is usually the last strategy tried because it is so counterintuitive for therapists. The strategy is incredibly simple: Therapists use less volume, less words, and less eye contact. This works on controlling and competitive children because when therapists whisper, it sounds like they are talking about a super special secret. This also works well on children with poor social interaction skills because it reduces the overall load of social interaction stimuli—verbal and body language—that they have to process. For most people, when they perceive that the other person does not understand them, their intuition is to increase the volume of their voice, use more words to explain themselves, and be more expressive to grab their attention. Those increases can work for people who are hard of hearing or inattentive, but they are counterproductive in our therapy situations.

Teddy was a 6-year-old boy who had been physically assaulted numerous times by his father. His parents were divorced and his mother was not available to be a caregiver because of her drug abuse. He was being cared for by his grandmother. Teddy was resistant to even come into the therapy room, so the therapist had negotiated to let him bring a few toys with him. When the therapist tried to direct his attention to the drawing exposure, he would deny that the event ever happened or argue about the first detail she brought up and involve himself with the toys. After several sessions of trying the time limit and the Tom Sawyer strategies, the therapist was out of tricks to try and finally attempted the "less is more" strategy. As Teddy was walking around the room, bouncing a rubber ball against the wall and trying to loudly convince the therapist to play with him, the therapist started to draw on the paper and whispered to herself.

"I'm going to draw the time that Dad hit Teddy in the back seat of the car."

Teddy continued to bounce the ball but he stopped talking.

"These are the wheels. Teddy is sitting in the back seat," she whispered as she drew the wheels and Teddy.

Teddy stopped bouncing the ball and walked over to look. "Hey," he said. "What's that?"

"That's Teddy sitting in the back of the yellow car. And here is Dad. He was angry." The therapist kept drawing without looking up at Teddy or offering to let him draw.

"Hey, I can do that," Teddy nearly demanded.

"Pick a crayon," the therapist whispered without stopping her drawing.

Teddy sat in the chair next to her and began drawing. The therapist continued to narrate in a whisper, "Teddy is in the back seat before that time Dad hit him. Dad is mad." At the same time she discreetly gathered up the toys off the table, collected them in a box, and slid them under the table.

Teddy drew details of the car rather than the actions of the physical assault, but he received the exposure through the visual reminder of the drawing and the therapist's narration of the event.

The Snack

The drawing exposure must be done on the table in the room. Uncooperative children are usually anywhere in the room except sitting at the table with the therapists. The snack is a simple trick to bring them to the table. Announce ever so casually that you think that now might be a good time for the snack. Leave the room briefly to retrieve the bag of chips and juice box and set them on the table. This intervention has the added advantage that while they eat the snack, their hands are tied up with the food and they stop talking while they chew.

All of these tricks, particularly the Tom Sawyer and "betcha can't" methods, work better if you do not oversell them. Children are inherently wired to detect trickery from adults. All of the strategies work best with a bit of "less is more" theatrics.

Safety Plans

The purpose of creating a safety plan is to give children a simple, memorized set of steps to follow if they are caught in a similar potentially traumatic situation again. The idea of a safety plan comes from the domestic violence field. Women who have been victims of domestic violence develop plans to escape to safety in the event that they feel threatened again; such a plan would include a hidden fund of cash and car keys and a friend to call. In the domestic violence field, safety plans are for the women, whereas in our treatment the safety plans are for the children.

The safety plan has two parts: (1) recognizing the danger signals and (2) enacting the action plan. Each plan ought to be individualized to the type of interpersonal trauma a child has experienced (e.g., domestic violence, physical abuse, community violence, natural disaster, dog attack).

Danger signals are cues that something bad is about to happen. For example, in cases of domestic violence, there is typically a build-up phase before Dads hit Moms, during which the perpetrator acts angry and mean. A lot of times both people yell, slam doors, and throw things before they get really, really mad. Following is a list of danger cues for different types of traumas:

Event	Danger Signals	Safety Plans
• Domestic violence	Door slammed; reddened face; things banged and thrown; yelling.	Tell Mom, "Daddy's angry." Older children may call 9-1-1.
• Sexual abuse	Left alone with older male.	Leave the room; find a safe adult.
• Community violence	Yelling, pushing, fighting.	Ask Mom to leave.
• MVA	No seat belt; going too fast; swerving; busy street.	Tell driver you are scared; ask driver to slow down; check seat belt.
• Dog attack	Growling; pulling at leash.	Tell Mom you're scared; keep away from dog.
• Natural disaster	Weather reports; warnings from the TV.	Pack special belongings in a suitcase; make plans for pets; store toys safely.

The ideal elements of an action plan for older children are to remove themselves from the danger and call for help if someone else (e.g., their mother) is in danger. This is not always possible for younger children who are more dependent on their caregivers.

The safety plan will be developed in Sessions 6–9. In Session 6, write out the tentative safety plan on the worksheet (Child Worksheet 6.2: My Safety Plan). In Session 7, use two puppets, one on each hand, to rehearse the safety plan. The purpose of the puppets is to make it more fun and to eventually engage the children more actively in rehearsing the plans. One puppet represents a child and the other represents a therapist. The therapist puppet narrates the occurrence of danger signals and asks the child puppet to recognize the danger signals and walk through the safety plan. Next, the children take over the child puppet and they walk through the plan again. In Session 8, the children take more responsibility for the puppets, either by taking control of both puppets or being the therapist puppet. After Session 8, the children and parents have a homework assignment to walk through the safety plan at home to work out any kinks. In Session 9, talk with the children about how the rehearsal of the safety plans went at home the previous week. If they found kinks in the plan, talk about how to troubleshoot and modify the plans.

Boundary Issues

Some caregivers are inappropriately intrusive of their children's personal boundaries for privacy and confidentiality. You will probably know fairly readily if a caregiver has that issue. For example, a caregiver may tell family members inappropriate things about what the child is doing in therapy. Or, the caregiver may try to get the child to do his or her homework and relaxation in front of other family members, even though the child is obviously embarrassed to do so. But even if the caregiver does not appear to have a boundary issue, we advocate to give all caregivers a preemptive spiel in Session 4 to prevent awkward moments in the future. This issue is repeated over the next several sessions, as needed.

Review Roadway Book

The two aims of this review are to provide one more iterative process for instilling the CBT techniques in the child, and to solidify the coherent narrative of the trauma experience.

The review is accomplished in steps over the final three sessions. In Session 10, review Sessions 1–6 in the Roadway Book. In Session 11, review Sessions 7–11. In Session 12, review Sessions 1–11. This gradual reiterative practice will give you and the family time to process any new distortions or difficulties that arise from the review process.

Conduct this review with the child and parent together. The goal is to reconsider the importance of every single page. It is a tall order for a child to be in charge of that task, and reading some of the words will be impossible for the younger children. Therefore, the therapist is ultimately in charge of exploring the pages and turning to the next one at an appropriate pace. Try to have the child remember what each page was about and what he or she learned. If the child can't, or won't, recall, the therapist must verbalize the material. Use lots of praise for children's accomplishments. This component should take 5–15 minutes per session.

Feasibility of Using CBT Techniques with Young Children

As noted earlier, using a 141-item treatment fidelity checklist, therapists' self-reports of fidelity to the protocol were excellent at 96.3%, and were corroborated by raters who independently scored nearly one-third of the sessions (Scheeringa, Weems, et al., 2011). Therapist fidelity to a protocol is the traditional method of substantiating that a standardized treatment was actually delivered. *However, fidelity only tracks what the therapists did.* Fidelity does not demonstrate the *feasibility* that the patients could actually comprehend, cooperate, and make effective use of the techniques. There is overlap between fidelity and feasibility, however. To some degree, patient cooperation is an implicit part of therapist fidelity, and effectiveness is an implicit part of treatment outcome measures, but it misses a dimension of how well the techniques were suited to the patients.

To capture this additional dimension of feasibility, we used another checklist to measure how well the children cooperated. We separately calculated the percentage of time that each task was accomplished, and these data were published with the original outcome data (Scheeringa, Weems, et al., 2011). The children were rated on the ability to complete 60 items over the 12 PPT sessions. The overall frequency of cooperation among children was 83.5%. The therapists made these ratings; an independent rater, who scored 30.7% of the treatment sessions, agreed with the therapists' ratings 96.2% of the time. The rater–therapists' interrater agreement kappa was substantial at 0.86.

The feasibility of the tasks was also calculated separately for 3-, 4-, 5-, and 6-year-old children. For example, the capacity to understand the concept of PTSD from verbal discussion in Session 1 for 3-year-old children was 0%. But when the concept was taught to them with the pictorial aid cartoons, 63% of them appeared to understand. In contrast, 92% of 6-year-old children appeared to understand the concept of PTSD from verbal discussion, and 100% grasped the concept with the pictorial aid cartoons. This pattern was typical for nearly all of the tasks. The 5- and 6-year-old children had an easier time grasping the concepts and performing the tasks, whereas the 3- and 4-year-old children had relatively more difficulty. It is worth noting that the difficulty was only relative. The 3- and 4-year-old children were able to eventually perform the key tasks in 100% of the cases.

A special note is made here about homework assignments. Prior to creating this manual, my experience with homework had been to assign it rather nonsystematically—that is, on an ad hoc, as-needed basis—and homework assignments were completed sporadically, at best. When we started testing this manual, we were quite uncertain as to whether parents would do these homework exposures with their children. It was enormously encouraging to see an overall completion percentage of 82%. These empirical data ought to give great confidence to therapists who have not used systematic homework assignments in their practices previously. Furthermore, our clinical experience with this manual indicated that the homework exposures were the more therapeutic compared to the in-office exposures. My speculation about this is that when children are in the office, the exposure is not quite real, and they can more easily avoid the intensity by distracting themselves or the therapists. With *in vivo* homework exposure, however, the exposure stimuli are quite real and unavoidable. It is during the *in vivo* exposures that all the elements of the therapy seem to come together: Children realize that they have fear reactions due to specific reminders, and that they have new relaxation skills that they can use.

Can Young Children Do Cognitive Therapy?

Doubts have been expressed as to whether young children can really do cognitive therapy. Grave and Blisset (2004) published a theoretical review that questioned whether CBT was developmentally appropriate for "young children" (Grave & Blissett, 2004). Interestingly, Grave and Blisset's definition of "young children" was 5–8 years; so we can infer that they would consider 3- and 4-year-old children even more inappropriate for CBT. Specifically, they questioned whether young children had the mature skills in causal reasoning, perspective taking, self-reflection, linguistic ability, and memory that were needed for the cognitive aspects of CBT.

Besides the empirical evidence we have gathered that this CBT is effective and the specific CBT techniques were feasible in 3- to 6-year-old children, we present additional conceptual considerations as to how cognitive therapy appears to be quite feasible with young children in this protocol:

- Because young children have probably never been asked to do this type of work before, they are potentially open to greater absolute change in their way of thinking than at any other age.
- In Session 1, their symptoms are given a name and put in a story form, which involves the cognitive tasks of self-reflection, autobiographical memory, and causal reasoning.
- In Session 3 their fears are placed in a bigger context of other feelings and other situations, which also involves the cognitive tasks of self-reflection, autobiographical memory, and causal reasoning.
- In Session 4, they are taught self-control with relaxation tools with the implicit message that these tools provide a change in locus of control within the self.
- In Sessions 5–11, the children complete exposure exercises. The protocol does not explicitly identify automatic negative thoughts, as do CBT protocols for depression, but it is often unavoidable during these narratives that involve thoughts of whether children felt appropriately or inappropriately safe, powerful, or effective. These types of thoughts are implicitly and sometimes explicitly addressed during the narratives.
- When repeatedly asked by therapists to engage in exposure and relaxation exercises, children receive an implicit message that control over anxiety is possible.
- In Session 11, children are asked to imagine themselves in future situations that may trigger anxiety. This is a purely cognitive task of perspective taking and causal reasoning.
- In Sessions 10–12, children review their drawing and homework sheets in their books, which involves the cognitive tasks of autobiographical memory and self-reflection.

Parent—Child Relational Considerations

Parents are heavily involved in this protocol because of logistical reasons. The parents are facilitators of the CBT techniques in that they provide history, interpret the children's body language, and help accomplish the homework tasks. Parents are viewed as complements that can make the CBT work better. It is tempting to view the parents as more than that, so it is important to make a distinction about what is empirically supported and what is not in regard to the impact of parenting behaviors. In short, parents are *not* viewed as causes of their children's symptoms, and they are not to be blamed for the symptoms.

We reviewed all of the studies that assessed the parent—child associations of problems following traumas that happened to the children (Scheeringa & Zeanah, 2001). Seventeen studies met our inclusion criteria that (1) the children had suffered DSM-IV-level life-threatening events, (2) the measures used in the study had to be standardized and replicable, and (3) the children and parents were assessed concurrently. A wide variety of constructs were measured and cannot all be reviewed in this space. In summary, all but one study found a significant association between worse parent outcome and worse child outcome. Many of the studies focused on PTSD symptoms and found that children with more symptoms or higher diagnosis rates of PTSD had parents with more symptoms or higher diagnosis rates of PTSD.

These data do not automatically imply that we need to treat the parent or the parent—child relationship. There are at least four theories to interpret this association.

1. The shared genetic history of parents and children may equally predispose them to developing symptoms following traumatic events. Moderate associations between specific genes and PTSD are gradually emerging, and it has been shown repeatedly in adults that the highly heritable pretrauma personality trait of neuroticism is a predisposing factor for PTSD (Fauerbach, Lawrence, Schmidt, Munster, & Costa, 2000). This research suggests that the genes that make parents vulnerable to develop PTSD are passed down to their children and make the children vulnerable to develop PTSD. In a prospective longitudinal assessment study of 1- to 6-year-old trauma-exposed children, we found a strong, positive correlation between children's and parents' PTSD, just like almost all prior studies, but parenting factors, measured in half a dozen different ways, explained very little of the variance in that relationship (Scheeringa, Myers, Putnam, & Zeanah, 2015). This finding suggests, by default, that shared genetic vulnerabilities may be a more likely explanation.

2. It may be that when both children and parents are more symptomatic, it is because the children suffered relatively more severe traumas, which vicariously traumatized the parents. Conversely, the children and parents who are both less symptomatic may have suffered less severe traumas. In other words, both children and parents reacted similarly to the severity of the traumas. The main drawback to that theory is that studies on PTSD have consistently shown that individual factors tend to be more important predictors of symptoms than degree of exposure (McFarlane, 1989), and the severity of exposure does not predict the majority of the variance in PTSD symptoms.

3. More disturbed parents may influence their children's symptoms. This theory suggests a directional relationship effect and has been the traditional "go-to" view for mental health professionals. That is, parent factors, acting through the parent–child relationship, have a causal impact on children's symptoms, at least for a subset of children. If the parent factors predated the traumatic events (e.g., harsh parenting), the parent factors may be called a *moderating*, or interaction, effect. If the parent factors were caused by the traumatic events (e.g., hostility toward their children as a result of the traumas), the parent factor may be called a *mediating* effect. At least one case study has suggested that parent–child relationship dynamics can hinder the successful adaptation of the child (MacLean, 1977, 1980). Case studies have also made it evident that caregivers do not have to be involved in the children's traumas at all to be symptomatic themselves and to appear important to treatment success (Pruett, 1979).

4. More disturbed children may influence their parents' symptoms. This is also a directional relationship effect but in the opposite direction from what professionals typically think. Parents may develop or maintain their own symptoms because they are distressed by their children's situations. In the Scheeringa et al. (2015) study, we also found that children with the most severe PTSD symptoms over time had parents who were more, not less, emotionally available and sensitive. This finding suggests that parents may have been reacting to their children's symptoms by becoming (appropriately) warmer and more sensitive to try to help their children cope. In addition, in the study that tested the PPT manual, we assessed the symptoms of the primary maternal caregivers with diagnostic interviews. The maternal symptoms of MDD significantly decreased from 4.2 (*SD* = 3.4) to 2.6 (*SD* = 2.7), but maternal PTSD symptoms, which were 9.3 (*SD* = 4.8) before PPT, remained high at 8.0 (*SD* = 4.8) after and did not significantly decrease. This finding suggests that the depression symptoms of mothers decreased as their children's PTSD symptoms decreased, and that mothers needed their own evidence-based treatment for their PTSD symptoms. When we asked mothers near the end of treatment whether they thought that they improved before their children improved or their children improved before they improved, nearly all of the mothers responded that their children improved first, and when they saw their children improve, that is when they could relax.

These are not mutually exclusive interpretations. All four interpretations may be true for one case, or each interpretation may be true for different subsets of dyads. The main point is to recognize the different possibilities, to not automatically blame the relationship, and to evaluate each patient on a case-by-case basis. The theories that appear to have the most traction, in my opinion, in the literature and in our experience are the first (shared genetic vulnerabilities) and the fourth (children influence parents) theories.

In a separate paper from that study that was published on the maternal symptoms, higher maternal depression did not have any impact on treatment gains immediately after the conclusion of therapy, but was associated with worsened children's PTSD symptoms when followed after 6 months (Weems & Scheeringa, 2013).

So how should the therapist best allocate time with the parents? The PPT protocol dictates that therapists spend at least part of every therapy session with the caregivers. The manual instructs therapists to be nondirective and to ask caregivers to reflect on the interactions they observed between their children and the therapists on the TV monitor. These reflections are viewed mainly as ways for caregivers to articulate what they have just been thinking about. Sometimes, although not usually, it is appropriate to steer these reflections to the caregivers' past individual experiences (i.e., past traumas); in that case, see the next section ("What If Parents Need Their Own Treatment?"). At other times, the manual instructs therapists to be directive and give advice.

The chief outcome for which we aim with parents is to facilitate the CBT tasks for the children. In some cases, caregivers have exceeded that aim and learned to alter their actual parenting behaviors. The mechanism by which this occurs appears to be from watching their children on the TV monitors and then reflecting about what they viewed with therapists. The parents who could engage in that level of reflection seem to be primed to do so, with minimal pressure needed from therapists. That is, the caregivers appeared to do the reflecting and mental processing alone while they were watching the sessions. They may have been provoked by therapists to think about salient issues, but they made changes in their perceptions, attitudes, and behaviors toward their children largely on their own. We have seen more than one "Aha!" moment occur when caregivers, because they were watching the sessions on TV, made a new connection to explain their children's behaviors. This is important to note because it runs contrary, for the most part, to traditional therapeutic wisdom that parents need coaching and/or psychodynamic interpretations of the meaning of their behaviors to make changes in their parenting.

An optional task is to ask about strong negative relational feelings in the dyad. Because of the unique salience of young children's dependence on their caregivers, negative feelings in the relationship may need to be detected and addressed. The child may have appropriately angry feelings at the mother, and the mother may have appropriately angry feelings at the perpetrator. The child may blame the mother for what happened. If this is realistic, some form of restitution, such as an apology or a sensitive, but simple, explanation may be needed. This kind of response can serve as validation for the young child. The parent may have angry and hurt feelings toward the perpetrator. For example, if the trauma was domestic violence, the mother may be angry with their spouse. Or, if the trauma was a dog mauling, the mother may be angry with the aunt who let the dog get loose. Although it is typically unrealistic to expect an apology from the other adult, it is a validating experience for the mother to discuss these feelings with the therapist and have them acknowledged as normal.

What If Parents Need Their Own Treatment?

In uncomplicated cases, caregivers are focused on the needs of their children. Complications do arise sometimes when the time spent with the caregivers is the most energy-consuming for therapists. If a caregiver is compelled to talk about his or her own intense symptoms and/or horrific childhood experiences, it may feel to the therapist as if the work with the child is being overshadowed. Remember that the child is not being short-changed because you always have individual time with the child.

The model of this manual is that the time reserved to spend alone with caregivers can be viewed as psychotherapy for them. Rather than refer caregivers out for their own therapies, you can attempt to treat caregivers in a limited fashion. This should be a supportive psychotherapy model, which includes active listening and advice giving. In my experience, this is easier said than done because child therapists seem to have an inherent bias to want to focus on the children and feel like they "off mission" if they are spending lots of time on the caregivers' issues. Bear in mind that many of these caregivers do not have anyone else to whom they can tell their stories, so I encourage you to listen and not cut them off, however tangentially related the conversation appears to their children.

Practical Matters

Each session lasts approximately 45–60 minutes. In Sessions 1, 2, and 12, the children and parents are together the entire sessions. In Sessions 3–11, half of that time is spent focused on the child and the second half with the mother. As noted, we have the mother watch the child's portion on TV in an adjacent room.

Take notes during sessions on specific words, phrases, or body language from the children that you do not understand. It is quite normal with this age group *not* to understand what the children are talking about. So, rather than "interrogate" them too much, which tends to be irritating because the children don't know how to express themselves more clearly, it is sometimes best to act as if you understand. Refer to your notes later in the session with the parents alone and *have the parents interpret* what the children were saying.

Do not jump forward over topics that are needed for later sessions. The sessions are arranged in the order they need to be followed for skills to develop that are needed for later sessions.

Generally, *do not move backward to repeat material*. If children do not appear to master techniques initially, it is not likely that they will master them any better simply by repetition. In fact, moving backward to repeat sessions will most likely be frustrating to children who are then unable to master the tasks a second time. The manual is designed with much repetition already built into the sequence of sessions, but with the repetition occurring in contexts that are increasingly salient to the children. As the office and homework exposures become increasingly anxiety-provoking, the techniques naturally become more salient to the children, and this salience usually provides the motivation and/or relevance that helps the children to grasp the techniques.

What If New Traumas Occur during Treatment?

Unfortunately, bad things do not happen at random. Children who have suffered traumatic events often live in families that disproportionately experience trauma and adversity (Nilsson, Gustafsson, & Svedin, 2012). We've developed the following guidelines to help structure a therapeutic response if a new trauma occurs in the middle of treatment. All of these may or may not be salient.

Mainly, step outside of the manual and spend a separate session (or more) on the new trauma to cover the following suggested topics:

- Get the details of what happened.
- Find out what the child actually saw, heard, or understands about it.
- Is there ongoing exposure or has the incident truly passed?
- Is the child truly not safe or does the child have an ongoing unrealistic sense of not being safe in the current environment? In other words, do you need to develop immediate safety and/or coping plans for real ongoing threats?
- Is the child repeatedly exposed to family or neighbors talking about it?
- Is the child repeatedly exposed to it daily from the television?
- Ask the mother what she has already been doing to help the child cope.
- If someone died, is a funeral planned?
- Is survival of the family an issue? That is, does the parent realistically need to be concerned primarily about shelter, food, and safety? If so, the daily nuances of parental sensitivity with children may be lost.
- Do one or more caregivers have PTSD symptomatology from the newest event?

The treatment plan for each situation can vary greatly depending on the unique circumstances. In general, a wait-and-watch approach for about 1 month is advocated to determine if new PTSD symptoms will endure from this new trauma (National Institute for Clinical Excellence, 2005). If symptoms endure after 1 month, then new events can be treated like old events and sessions used to tell the narrative, incorporate events into the old stimulus hierarchy or create a separate one, and conduct office and homework exposures.

The question may arise as to whether treatment for PTSD should stop when there are ongoing threats in the environment. The logic would be that when children are stressed by ongoing threats in their environments, the additional stress of exposure therapy could push the children beyond their emotional limits. The principle for managing this additional stress, however, is the same as the principle for determining how aggressively to pursue exposures. Each step taken is a consensual, negotiated, incremental action, and the stress on the children is constantly reevaluated. In that sense, there is no known absolute contraindication to conducting therapy during ongoing stress. Certainly, exposure-type therapy adds to one's overall stress level, at least temporarily, but the treatment is also quite likely to be the main means of relieving the stress. Furthermore, one must ask, if exposure-type therapy is not conducted, then what does one do? Does one simply not provide a known evidence-based therapy for an undetermined period of time for an ongoing life circumstance that may never change?

Therapist Prerequisites

Therapist prerequisites are few and of minimal difficulty to achieve. The only prerequisite for a therapist is that he or she is a licensed psychiatrist, psychologist, social worker, or other type of counselor who must be willing to follow a structured protocol.

Optional background that can be helpful includes prior didactics and experience in the implementation of these techniques:

- CBT in children.
- Treatment of PTSD in children.
- Treatment of PTSD in adults.
- Knowledge of parent–child relational issues in preschool children.

How Closely Should You Follow the Manual?: Some Thoughts on Implementation of Evidence-Based Treatments in Community Clinics

I personally believe that one of the factors that prevents clinicians from adopting evidence-based treatments is that they are too hard on themselves. They have concerns that they will not be able to perform the treatment techniques as well and as cleanly as the techniques are described in manuals. Because they do not want to do something poorly, they do not attempt it all and find other rationalizations for why a structured or manual-based therapy will not work.

I think it is useful to think of *high fidelity* and *medium fidelity*. In high fidelity, therapists follow the manual closely—very closely. In medium fidelity, therapists commit themselves more to making the attempts, expecting imperfection and mistakes, rather than hold expectations of perfect execution.

A fidelity measure—the Fidelity and Achievement ChecklisT (FACT)—is provided in Appendix 2. Therapists should fill out this measure after each session. Therapists rate themselves on whether or not they followed the manual with high fidelity or medium fidelity. In addition, therapists rate the achievements of the children—that is, whether children were able to cooperate and/or complete their tasks.

Cheat Sheets

Therapists cannot memorize all of the manual tasks, so they ought to refer to the manual frequently during sessions. An alternative to the manual is to have *cheat sheets* on the table in the therapy room during sessions to which they can frequently refer. Sample cheat sheets for each session are provided in Appendix 3. In my experience, I have found that individual therapists prefer their own personalized cheat sheets, and it is anticipated that the cheat sheets provided in Appendix 3 will serve as templates for others to create their own.

CHAPTER 2

Assessment

What Are Traumas for Young Children?

Since the publication of the *Diagnostic and Statistical Manual of Mental Disorders, Third Edition, Revised* (DSM-III-R; American Psychiatric Association, 1987), the definition of trauma for PTSD has been clearly operationalized as *life-threatening* or a threat of serious harm. This clarity was maintained through the fourth and fifth editions of the DSM (DSM-IV and DSM-5). These types of events include, but are not limited to, sexual abuse, physical abuse, witnessing domestic violence, frightening medical procedures, dog attacks, disasters, war, severe motor vehicle accidents, and other types of accidental injuries. Yet, trauma is in the eye of the beholder, particularly for young children. A dog attack is truly life-threatening to a 3-year-old child, but the same dog attack may not be to a 15-year-old adolescent.

What makes something life-threatening or a threat of serious harm? The content of the events, of course, plays the largest role, and the content of events that are life-threatening or a threat to serious harm is rather straightforward: severe motor vehicle accidents, physical abuse, sexual abuse, witnessing domestic violence, floods, tornados, earthquakes, and missile strikes, just to name some of the most common events. Two other key aspects of events that have been supported by research are that the events are *sudden* and produce a *sense of panic* in the persons. The death of a parent that is expected after a 2-year-long battle with cancer and occurs without gruesome incident is typically not perceived as an event that can cause PTSD. But the death of a parent that occurred suddenly from a heart attack in the living room in front of the children is more likely to cause PTSD.

Attempts have been made to broaden the definition of trauma to include non-life-threatening events such as bullying, property crime (Finkelhor, Ormrod, & Turner, 2007), out-of-home placement, parental drug abuse (Ford, Connor, & Hawke, 2009), neglect, and emotional abuse (Cloitre et al., 2009; Hickman et al., 2012; Hodges et al., 2013). These types of non-life-threatening events have been associated with internalizing or externalizing problems, but there is no evidence that these types of events lead to PTSD. For those types of non-life-threatening events to cause PTSD, some aspect of the events would have to appear life-threatening to the children. For example, a 5-year-old child who experienced out-of-home placement witnessed her father fight with the police when they came to remove her from the home. Her father was bloodied, handcuffed, taken away, and she thought his life was in danger. The placement in another home need not necessarily appear to be life-threatening, but the related incident of the fight between her father and the police by itself appeared life-threatening.

Attempts have also been made to broaden the concept of a posttraumatic syndrome beyond PTSD to various syndromes called "symptom complexity" (Cloitre et al., 2009) and "developmental trauma disorder" (van der Kolk, 2005). At this point, these speculative syndromes lack preliminary validity data and have not yet achieved face validity (Scheeringa, 2015). In addition, it has not been documented that PTSD fails to adequately represent the signs and symptoms of chronically and repeatedly traumatized youngsters (Roth, Newman, Pelcovitz, van der Kolk, & Mandel, 1997).

Assessment of PTSD Is More Difficult Compared to Other Disorders

The right treatment must be paired to the right diagnosis, which hinges on an accurate assessment. There are multiple considerations that make the accurate assessment of posttraumatic stress symptoms and the diagnosis of PTSD quite difficult. These considerations add time, tension, or a degree of difficulty to the assessment encounters.

1. PTSD requires an etiological event. Before one can even ask about symptoms of PTSD, one must ask about traumatic events. Furthermore, because it is very common that children have experienced more than one traumatic event (Copeland, Keeler, Angold, & Costello, 2007), one ought to ask about all possible traumatic experiences. Eliciting this information can add a substantial amount of time to an assessment for a busy clinician.

2. There are 20 possible symptoms in the PTSD DSM-5 criteria. This is more than double the number found in nearly all other disorders. I have previously published data on how long it took to interview caregivers about a variety of disorders using a standardized diagnostic interview (Scheeringa, 2011):

- 52.4 minutes for PTSD.
- 25.6 minutes for MDD.
- 13.3 minutes for ADHD.
- 10.3 minutes for ODD.
- 8.0 minutes for phobias.
- 6.5 minutes for SAD.
- 4.3 minutes for generalized anxiety disorder (GAD).

The data were from a study of 3- to 6-year-old trauma-exposed children, so the times may not be representative of the entire clinical population, but are probably pretty close for clients with PTSD. The time can be greatly reduced, however, by starting with self-administered questionnaires instead of interviews.

3. Symptoms must be dated by time of onset. In order to know for sure that symptoms started following traumatic events and are truly PTSD symptoms, as opposed to preexisting non-PTSD symptoms, dates of symptom onset must be collected—which adds more time to the assessment.

4. Memories of traumatic events are unpleasant. The nature of memories of traumatic events makes the assessment of all PTSD symptoms distressing usually, and can lead to an underestimation of symptoms. In particular, two of the symptoms concern the avoidance of reminders of past events. When asked about symptoms, respondents may reply, "I don't want to talk about it," which puts up a roadblock that sensitive clinicians fear to cross. Or, they may respond, "I don't think about it," which initially sounds like the absence of symptoms but may actually be an endorsement of avoidance symptoms (Cohen & Scheeringa, 2009).

5. Avoidance can be perceived as normative instead of as symptomatic. A common misunderstanding of PTSD symptoms occurs around the decision to regard the avoidance of reminders of past traumas as a normative adaptation or a maladaptive symptom. For example, a 5-year-old girl was hit by a car while crossing a street. Afterward, she refused to cross streets if moving cars were in sight and crossed with great reluctance even when no cars were in sight. Often, these behaviors are perceived (incorrectly) as good judgment—that is, she learned from experience. What this perception fails to acknowledge is that whereas caution is a normative reaction for children when crossing busy streets, fear is not. Avoidant behaviors that are coupled with fear reactions are not normative reactions. Disentangling these issues adds time to the assessments.

6. Many PTSD symptoms are highly internalized, which makes them difficult for children to express with their still-developing language capacities and difficult for parents to observe. Internalized symptoms include avoidance of internalized reminders (e.g., efforts to distract oneself when memories of traumatic events intrude into one's mind) of past traumas, certain types of psychological distress in response to reminders of traumas, physiological reactivity to reminders of traumas, dissociative experiences, intrusive recollections, and perhaps nightmares. Additional questions and time are needed to probe for these symptoms.

7. Because most persons have never had PTSD, caregivers may have no common frame of reference from which to report on their children's feelings. In contrast, nearly everyone intuitively understands sadness, hyperactivity, and defiance, which make depression, ADHD, and ODD relatively easier to detect. Additional questions and time are needed for the PTSD assessment because the interviewer often must educate the respondent about each symptom before asking about it.

8. Many PTSD symptoms manifest differently at different developmental stages. For example, the symptom of intrusive recollections is manifest by school-age children almost entirely by verbalizations, but is manifest by many preschool-age children as

reenactments in their play that do not depend so heavily on verbalizations. Avoidance behaviors, restricted range of affect, diminished interest in activities, detachment from loved ones, difficulty concentrating, and irritability/outbursts of anger may also have systematic differences in presentations by age. Multiple ways of asking about a symptom may be needed—which, again, requires additional time and effort.

9. When asking questions about traumatic events, interviewers often feel concerned that they will cause misery and melancholy for the respondents, which leads interviewers to skip such questions out of concerns for their own or their clients' distress. Such concerns are largely unwarranted, as clinical experience and research data have converged on the conclusion that these questions rarely cause marked distress. In a sample that was recruited to represent the U.S. population of 10- to 17-year-old children and adolescents, telephone interviews were conducted with 2,312 youth. All participants received an enhanced version of the Juvenile Victimization Questionnaire. Only 4.6% reported being at all upset by answering survey questions, and only 0.3% (seven children) would not participate again. Of the seven who would not participate again, only one cited the nature of the questions as the reason for no further participation (another reason included the time commitment; Finkelhor, Vanderminden, Turner, Hamby, & Shattuck, 2014). In my experience, my colleagues and I have interviewed over 500 trauma-exposed caregivers and children of all ages and seen most of them repeatedly in longitudinal or treatment settings, and they have rarely appeared markedly distressed. Most of them find it reassuring that a professional has taken an interest in their personal stories. When they do appear markedly distressed, it is obvious quite early on and the interviews can be easily stopped.

What Do We Know about Assessing PTSD in Young Children?

When PTSD was first included as a diagnostic category in DSM-III (American Psychiatric Association, 1980), there were few data available on children younger than 18 years old, and almost no data on children younger than 12 years old. That situation has changed dramatically, as much research has been conducted on PTSD in young children from 1995 to the present in an effort to establish diagnostic validity, improve assessment techniques, and develop treatment protocols.

Ten studies have examined PTSD symptoms in young children, using developmentally sensitive criteria (Bogat, DeJonghe, Levendosky, Davidson, & von Eye, 2006; Ghosh-Ippen, Briscoe-Smith, & Lieberman, 2004; Levendosky, Huth-Bocks, Semel, & Shapiro, 2002; Meiser-Stedman et al., 2008; Ohmi et al., 2002; Scheeringa et al., 1995, 2001, 2003; Scheeringa & Zeanah, 2008; Stoddard et al., 2006), compared to two such studies in school-age and adolescent children (Meiser-Stedman et al., 2008; Scheeringa, Wright, Hunt, & Zeanah, 2006), so that the field of PTSD is in an unusual position in which diagnostic validity has been studied more meticulously in young children than in school-age and adolescent children.

Even in the first study of diagnostic validity in very young children, it was clear from reviewing signs and symptoms of highly symptomatic, traumatized young children that they could not meet the algorithm for the DSM-IV diagnosis of PTSD (Scheeringa et al.,

1995). This was largely due to the requirement for three avoidance and numbing items. The cluster of seven avoidance and numbing items was also the most internalized of the three PTSD clusters. If the requirement for the numbing and avoidance items was lowered to one item, then young children could qualify for the diagnosis at reasonable rates (Scheeringa et al., 1995, 2001, 2003).

When researchers used developmentally sensitive assessment methods and diagnostic criteria, they have found PTSD to be common in young children following traumatic events. The rates of PTSD were 38% following war-related trauma (Feldman & Vengrober, 2011), 17% following the World Trade Center disaster (DeVoe, Bannon, & Klein, 2006), 10% following motor vehicle accidents (Meiser-Stedman et al., 2008), 13% following burns (De Young et al., 2012; Graf et al., 2011), 25% following a gas explosion in Japan (Ohmi et al., 2002), and 26% following exposure to domestic violence (Levendosky et al., 2002; Scheeringa et al., 2003). The rates are much higher, 60–69%, in trauma-exposed clinic samples (Scheeringa et al., 1995, 2001).

Based on the empirical findings from these studies, we proposed several iterations of new criteria for the diagnosis of PTSD in very young children (Scheeringa et al., 1995, 2003). The most significant proposed change was to reduce the number of avoidance and numbing items that are required from three symptoms to one symptom. Note that lowering the threshold for criterion C has been suggested even for adults because highly symptomatic and impaired adults could not be given the diagnosis if they had only two but not three criterion C symptoms (Kilpatrick & Resnick, 1993).

Changes in wording of four items were also proposed to improve the face validity of the items:

1. For the symptom "recurrent and intrusive distressing recollections of the event," we proposed to include a note that the distress may not be obvious. For example, a 4-year-old boy who had witnessed severe domestic violence perpetrated on his mother by his father announced to the cashier at the grocery store, "My daddy hit my mommy." He did not appear to be distressed, and even appeared somewhat eager to talk about it.

2. Change the wording of "markedly diminished interest or participation in significant activities" to reflect the significant activities of young children, which are play, social interactions, and daily routines. The same 4-year-old boy refused to go outside or ride his bike, and paid attention to TV for only a few minutes. He did not have school, work, sports, or hobbies on which to be judged.

3. Change the wording of "feeling of detachment or estrangement from others" (a highly internalized phenomenon) to "social withdrawal," which is more behavioral and observable. A 5-year-old boy who had several life-threatening experiences during Hurricane Katrina had been close with his mother's girlfriend and her twin boys that were his same age. After the disaster, he was not interested in seeing his mom's girlfriend or in playing with the twins.

4. Change the wording of "irritability or outbursts of anger" to include new or extreme temper tantrums. The same 5-year-old boy became easily annoyed and irritable at minor provocations after the disaster.

The latest iteration generated from this highly empirical process is summarized in Table 2.1. These suggestions were accepted in a new diagnosis in the DSM-5 termed "PTSD in children 6 years and younger" (American Psychiatric Association, 2013). This diagnosis represents a landmark for the DSM-5 because it is the first ever developmental subtype of a major psychiatric disorder. Using alternative diagnostic criteria that are very similar to the new DSM-5 disorder, eight studies have calculated rates of PTSD in head-to-head comparisons with the DSM-IV criteria (Egger et al., 2006; Levendosky et al., 2002; Meiser-Stedman et al., 2008; Ohmi et al., 2002; Scheeringa et al., 1995, 2001, 2003, 2012). The alternative criteria always diagnosed more cases than the DSM-IV criteria and demonstrated greater diagnostic validity (Scheeringa, Zeanah, & Cohen, 2011). For example, in a sample of 2- to 6-year-old children recruited from a nursery school after a gas explosion in the building, 0% could be diagnosed with PTSD by the DSM-IV criteria, but 25% could be diagnosed with the alternative criteria.

It is worth noting, however, that the new DSM-5 disorder includes a new symptom, described by confusing terminology, for which there is no empirical support. The new symptom is "increased frequency of negative emotional states (e.g., fear, guilt, sadness, shame, or confusion)." The PTSD criteria already contained symptoms reflecting negative emotional states such as psychological distress in response to reminders of the trauma and avoidance of reminders of the trauma. Internal or external reminders trigger

TABLE 2.1. Proposed Criteria for PTSD in Young Children

Item	Change from DSM-IV
Reexperiencing symptoms: Require one out of five possible symptoms.	
• Intrusive recollections not required to be distressing	Not required to be distressing.
• Nightmares	
• Dissociation	
• Psychological distress at reminders of the trauma	
• Physiological distress at reminders of the trauma	
Avoidance and numbing symptoms: Require one instead of three symptoms.	
• Avoid thoughts, feelings, conversations that resemble the trauma	
• Avoid activities, places, people that resemble the trauma	
• Diminished interests emphasize play constriction	Includes emphasis on play as an important interest.
• Socially withdrawn behavior	Wording is more behavioral, less internalized.
• Restricted affect	
• Do not include two symptoms: inability to recall trauma and sense of foreshortened future.	
Increased arousal: Require two out of five possible symptoms.	
• Sleep difficulty	
• Irritability, including excessive temper tantrums	Includes temper tantrums.
• Concentration difficulty	
• Hypervigilance	
• Exaggerated startle response	

these existing symptoms. The wording of the new symptom, as "increased frequency of negative emotional states," contains nothing to indicate how it differs from the negative emotional states of the previously identified symptoms. The only aspect that could distinguish the new symptom from the prior symptoms is that internal or external reminders of the traumas do not trigger the new symptom—but the new symptom is worded in such a vague fashion that it is not clear. Emotional distress from triggered reminders or avoidance could well be coded inaccurately as "negative emotional states" when respondents are unaware of the triggers (e.g., caregivers as respondents), or when interviewers do not adequately probe for the existence of triggers—both common problems that have been previously noted (Cohen & Scheeringa, 2009). Indeed, in the first test of this new symptom, 95% of those with it also had at least one of the symptoms in which negative emotion is expressed in response to a trauma trigger. It seems possible that negative emotions from triggered trauma reactions were being double-coded as "negative emotional states" (Scheeringa et al., 2012). This study did not assess the negative emotional states of guilt, shame, and confusion; however, it is not clear that these would have changed the results substantially. These emotions are highly internalized phenomena that are difficult for young children to verbalize, if at all, and difficult for caregivers to infer from behavioral observations.

One additional note is that our research has identified four symptoms that are common in young children following traumas: (1) regression in skills (e.g., verbal skills, dressing skills, and toileting), (2) new onset of separation anxiety, (3) new onset of physical aggression, and (4) new onset of fears of things not related to the trauma (e.g., going to the bathroom alone, and the dark). Although including these items in the diagnostic criteria does not increase the diagnostic sensitivity (Scheeringa et al., 2003), they may be useful when educating caregivers about posttraumatic reactions and as items on treatment outcome measures.

Symptomatic and Impaired, but Not Diagnosed

Like any medical or psychiatric diagnosis in which symptomatology exists along a continuum of severity (Angold, Costello, Farmer, Burns, & Erkanli, 1999), a PTSD diagnostic dichotomy underestimates the number of children with symptoms and related functional impairment. In our 2-year prospective study of 1- to 6-year-old trauma-exposed children, significantly more children at baseline were impaired in at least one domain of functioning (48.9%) than had the full diagnosis of PTSD (23.4%) ($n = 47$); the gap was even greater after 2 years (74.3% impaired compared to 22.9% diagnosed; $n = 35$) (Scheeringa et al., 2005). Similar types of results have been found in 7- to 14-year-old children (Carrion, Weems, Ray, & Reiss, 2002).

Recognition of children who are impaired but not diagnosed is important because current practice parameters recommend that children with clinically significant impairing levels of PTSD symptoms, regardless of diagnostic status, should be provided with evidence-supported treatment options (Cohen & the American Academy of Child and Adolescent Psychiatry, 1998).

Assessment Measures

There are two options for the assessment of PTSD symptoms: (1) self-administered questionnaires that the caregivers complete on their own or (2) interviews conducted by trained interviewers. A self-administered questionnaire has the advantage that it requires less time, usually about 10–15 minutes, which also makes it easier to readminister to track progress (see Table 2.2). This method is usually the overwhelming choice for busy practitioners. An interview, in contrast, can take an average of over 50 minutes (Scheeringa, 2011), but it has the advantage of being more accurate. The reexperiencing and avoidance items are routinely misunderstood (see Chapter 1), and an interviewer can educate the respondent about the items before asking about them. This is usually the choice for small- to medium-size research studies. Questions posed to children younger than 7 years of age have proven infeasible and of no additional value (Scheeringa et al., 2001). Although some effort has been directed toward development of measures for young children as respondents (Measelle, Ablow, Cowan, & Cowan, 1998), all known diagnostic measures are limited to children 7 years of age and older.

Self-Administered Questionnaires

Young Child PTSD Checklist

I created the Young Child PTSD Checklist (YCPC; Scheeringa, 2010) because there were no self-administered questionnaires that mapped straightforwardly onto the PTSD criteria for young children. The measure includes a trauma events screen with a menu of eight possible types of traumatic events. It is the only known questionnaire that collects information for each type of event data on the age of the first traumatic event, the age of the last traumatic event, and an estimate of the number of times a trauma has happened. The 23 symptom-related questions have been updated to reflect changes in DSM-5. In addition, I included four associated symptoms that have been shown empirically to follow an experience of trauma in young children (physical aggression, separation anxiety, regression in developmental skills, and fears of new situations not related to the trauma) (Scheeringa et al., 1995, 2001, 2003). There are six items on functional impairment. Each item is rated on a 0–4 Likert scale, so the range of symptom scores is 0–92 and the range of impairment scores is 0–24. Although there is the limitation that psychometric data on construct validity and test–retest reliability have not been reported (these are currently being collected), these issues are not of great concern for measures that

TABLE 2.2. Pros and Cons of Self-Administered Questionnaire versus Interview for the Assessment of PTSD

	Pros	Cons
Self-administered questionnaire	• Time requirement is about 10 minutes. • Easier to re-administer to track progress.	• Less accurate. • Interviewer not available to explain items.
Interview	• More accurate. • Interviewer can explain items.	• Time requirement is about 50 minutes.

map straightforwardly onto diagnostic criteria. Construct validation psychometrics are more important for measures of latent constructs that cannot be operationally and wholly defined by a specific set of questions, such as IQ and personality. The YCPC is free and available at *www.infantinstitute.org/measures.htm*.

Trauma Symptom Checklist for Young Children

The Trauma Symptom Checklist for Young Children (TSCYC; Briere, 2005) is a 90-item parent-report checklist for assessing posttrauma reactions in 3- to 12-year-olds. Each item is rated on a 1–4 Likert scale. The TSCYC produces nine clinical scales—Posttraumatic Stress–Intrusion, Posttraumatic Stress–Avoidance, Posttraumatic Stress–Arousal, Sexual Concerns, Anxiety, Depression, Dissociation, and Anger/Aggression—and provides a tentative PTSD diagnosis with the summary Post-Traumatic Stress–Total scale. The measure also contains two validity scales to check for overreporting (Atypical Response) or underreporting (Response Level). Norms are based on gender and age breakdowns of 3–4, 5–9, and 10–12. The TSCYC has correctly classified 95.7% of participants without a PTSD diagnosis (specificity); its limitations include that it correctly classified only 54.5% of participants with a PTSD diagnosis (sensitivity) (Pollio, Glover-Orr, & Wherry, 2008). Other limitations include low reliabilities of the underreporting scale (only fair) and the overreporting scale (poor) (Briere et al., 2001). The measure is not free and is relatively lengthy. The validation studies have grouped 3- to 12-year-old children and have not focused on 3- to 6-year-olds.

For a more detailed review of other measures for this population, see De Young et al. (in press). Of particular note is that the Child Behavior Checklist for Ages 1½–5 (CBCL/1½–5; Achenbach & Rescorla, 2000) cannot be recommended for this population despite the CBCL being one of the most widely used measures of emotional and behavioral functioning. Studies have created an ad hoc PTSD subscale from a subset of items and suggested using the CBCL as a screen for PTSD (Wolfe, Gentile, & Wolfe, 1989), but the CBCL was not designed to measure PTSD and lacks any symptoms that are unique to PTSD (Dehon & Scheeringa, 2006; Levendosky et al., 2002).

Interviews

For the most accurate information on traumatic events and PTSD symptoms, a diagnostic interview must be used. Only in an interview can the interviewer educate the respondent about the items and clarify answers with follow-up probes. I created the Diagnostic Infant and Preschool Assessment (DIPA) in 2004 specifically for this purpose. The DIPA includes modules for 15 disorders, including PTSD; has been updated for DSM-5; and is freely available at *www.infantinstitute.org/measures.htm*.

In a psychometric validation study (Scheeringa & Haslett, 2010), the caregivers of 50 outpatients, ages 1–6 years, were interviewed twice by trained interviewers using the DIPA, once by a clinician, and once by a research assistant, concerning eight disorders (PTSD, MDD, ADHD–inattentive subtype, ADHD–hyperactive/impulsive subtype,

ODD, SAD, GAD, and obsessive–compulsive disorder [OCD]). The median test–retest intraclass correlation was .69, the mean was .61, and the values ranged from .24 to .87. The median test–retest kappa was 0.53, the mean was 0.52, and the values ranged from 0.38 to 0.66. There were no differences by duration between interviews. Concurrent criterion validity showed good agreement between the instrument and DSM-based CBCL scales when the DSM-based scales were matched well to the disorder (ADHD–inattentive subtype, ADHD–hyperactive/impulsive subtype, and ODD).

Although the DIPA is free and clinicians with any level of experience are encouraged to use it, specific training and techniques are needed for best results, particularly for the PTSD module (Scheeringa, 2011). As noted earlier, most caregivers have never had PTSD, so they have no common frame of reference from which to report on their children's PTSD symptoms. As noted previously, although most everyone intuitively understands sadness, hyperactivity, and defiance, most everyone does not intuitively understand many of the PTSD symptoms, so interviewers must educate respondents about these symptoms before asking about each one. For example, interviewers must probe further than simply asking "Does your child get distressed when something reminds him [her] about the trauma?" If the respondents reply, "No," then the interviewers must provide possible examples. If a child's trauma was domestic violence, the interviewer might ask, "What about if another adult starts to argue with you?" If a child's trauma was a motor vehicle accident, the interviewer might ask, "What happens when she [he] has to ride in a car again?" Concerns that this type of interviewing is "leading the witness" are generally unfounded. Concerns about fabricating symptoms are justified for malingerers and adults seeking financial gain. Nevertheless, the DIPA has a failsafe strategy that every "Yes" answer must be supported by a specific example that is convincing to the interviewers.

Oppositional Defiant Behavior

Studies on disorders comorbid with PTSD in young children have shown that ODD is often the most common disorder that develops following trauma after PTSD. In our study of 62 1- to 6-year-old children, of those with PTSD, 75% also had ODD (SAD was second most common at 63%) (Scheeringa et al., 2003). These findings converge nicely with our clinical experience in which caregivers seem more likely to bring their children for treatment because they are concerned about their disruptive and externalizing behaviors than their anxious and internalized behaviors. These disruptive types of behaviors tend to cause the most functional impairment in home, day care, and other settings.

We created Session 2 of the manual to proactively address these disruptive behaviors. Chapter 1 described how discipline plans are developed to target children's oppositional and defiant behaviors. Although the caregivers usually bring these up spontaneously during the intake sessions, the manual provides step-by-step instructions in Session 2 on how to ask about and clearly operationalize these problems. If clinicians want a standardized measure to assess the severity of these symptoms and/or to track progress over time, the Swanson, Nolan, and Pelham (SNAP) scale is a widely used measure that maps directly onto the symptoms of ODD (Kollins et al., 2006) and is free from many sites on the Internet.

Grief

Also in Session 2 of the manual, plans to address grief are developed if traumas involved loss of loved ones, and grief reactions continue to be problematic. The manual provides specific suggestions about how to assess for and treat grief reactions. These methods are often sufficient, but for a more detailed guidance on dealing with grief, an excellent resource is Salloum (1998).

The Intake Assessment before Session 1

Before starting Session 1 of the treatment manual, an intake assessment obviously needs to be conducted to determine diagnosis, the type of treatment that is needed, and gather essential background information. We typically conduct an initial assessment that is spent mostly on obtaining history from caregivers. The young children are often present because these children are usually not in school and caregivers do not have babysitters. The children are either in the room with the clinicians and caregivers, entertained with toys, or playing while supervised in an adjacent room if an assistant is available. If it can be arranged, it is usually preferable to meet with caregivers alone in order to discuss difficult topics privately. These topics include marriage or boyfriend history, siblings, who else lives in the home, employment, day care or preschool, detailed story of the traumatic event(s), and medical issues.

We then conduct a second assessment that involves the children mostly, which we call the "Getting to Know You" session. This time is spent engaging with the children to build a working relationship. Games and toys are used, but care should be taken to avoid having multiple toys in the room because the therapy is not conducted with toys in the room. If the children have a lot of toys to pick from at the first session, they will be disappointed at later sessions when there are no toys. Follow the child's lead and allow him or her to get to know you just by being with you a bit. If the child doesn't want to separate from the mother, have the mother stay in the room while you play. This session can also be used to follow up with questions for the caregivers that you did not have time for in the first assessment session.

PART II

Treatment Manual

Psychoeducation

✓ *Get acquainted.*

✓ *Provide education about PTSD.*

✓ *Provide overview of the 12 sessions.*

✓ *Provide motivation/compliance preparation.*

About This Session

The child and parent are seen together for the entire session.

Materials

- Candy and snacks: The ground rules about candy and snacks need to be covered. Small, soft candy will be offered once at the beginning. Snacks (chips and juice) will be offered after the child's session, to be consumed while the child plays during the parent's session. Giving the snack during their session actually helps to keep some children "at the table," literally, and increases their compliance. However, snacks are not to be used as a reward or withheld as an enticement.

- Two three-prong binders for the child's book and homework.

- Stickers for the book cover and for homework sheets.

- Markers.

- Handout sheets for the Roadway Book.

- Outline of the 12 sessions in Parent Handout 1.1.

- Parent Handout 1.2 on PTSD and common symptoms from trauma.

- Illustrations of PTSD symptoms.

Conducting the Session

Parent and Child Together

Introduction and Rules

With both mother and child in the room, explain that this is the beginning of therapy and that there are some ground rules to cover that include a typical sequence of events for every session: (1) The child receives a piece of candy, (2) the work is focused on child, (3) the work is focused on the parent while the child snacks, and (4) the homework is planned with the parent and child together.

If the child is not interested in the candy, do not make it an issue. Make it clear that the candy will be put away (out of sight) and unavailable for the rest of this session. For children who try to take more than one piece of candy, don't offer a dish full of candy; offer two choices or even just one.

Describe the Purpose of the Sessions

Next, give the mother the outline of the treatment: Parent Handout 1.1: Overview of the 12 Treatment Sessions).* Because young children often associate doctor offices with vaccination shots, explain to the child that you don't give shots in your office. Then make it clear at the start that both the child and the caregiver are seeing you to deal with the trauma and the symptoms of PTSD by acquiring some tools to help them feel better. Tell them that you and they will meet 12 times.

Describe PTSD

Give Parent Handout 1.2: Posttraumatic Stress Disorder (PTSD) to the caregiver. Briefly describe how we know that traumas can cause symptoms in people. Define a life-threatening trauma, using examples that are relevant for adults and different ones for little children to give them perspective.

Next, introduce the terms *posttraumatic stress disorder* and *PTSD* for the caregivers. For the children, reframe this term as "your scary feelings" or "your scary thoughts." We've found that the acronym *PTSD* is too abstract for young children.

Now describe the different kinds of symptoms, referring to Parent Handout 1.2. Avoid going through all 17 PTSD symptoms verbally as this is too much information to process. The handout has these details for parents to read later. Focus instead on the three types of symptom clusters and use a made-up example that is different from their real trauma to illustrate.

---

*See Part III (pp. 125–158) and Appendices 1–3 (pp. 159–212) for all reproducible materials.

Example of Defining Trauma and PTSD: Andrew

Andrew is a 4-year, 1-month-old boy who survived Hurricane Katrina in New Orleans. The therapist has just briefly established with the child and mother that the "scary thing that happened to you was the hurricane." The therapist is directing comments primarily to the caregiver at this point.

THERAPIST: When something scary like that happens, children and adults can experience what's called *trauma*. This trauma is something that scared you, or perhaps someone you love died or got hurt really badly. There are different types of trauma. A hurricane can cause trauma, and so can car crashes, physical abuse, and dog bites. Any type of life-threatening event can cause trauma. Some time after the trauma has occurred, some people get posttraumatic stress disorder, which has three main types of problems: reexperiencing, numbness and avoidance, and hyperarousal. So with reexperiencing, it's things like . . . (*turning toward the child*) Hey, Andrew, have you ever had a nightmare?

ANDREW: Yeah.

THERAPIST: What do you have nightmares about?

ANDREW: The dark.

THERAPIST: So (*turning toward the mom*) nightmares and sometimes daydreams really upset Andrew if they remind him of the storm.

MOM: Like rain, huh? You don't like it when it rains?

ANDREW: No.

THERAPIST: Another type of problem that can come with trauma is numbing and avoidance—kind of shutting down. People with this kind of problem try to stay away from anything that makes them think about it. They might be more withdrawn, might not look so happy any more. (*pause*) The third type of problem is called *hyperarousal*. Kids who have been traumatized usually get really wound up and have difficulty sleeping and difficulty concentrating; they are easily irritated, have temper tantrums, and are generally more aggressive, jumpy, and scared. These are the three main types of symptoms for posttraumatic stress.

Next, use the illustrations of some of the PTSD symptoms (see Appendix 1) to help illustrate these concepts to the child. Typically, three illustrations are enough to show the child. Let the child name the boy or girl in the illustration (the potential problem with you picking the name is that you may inadvertently pick a name of someone with whom the child had a bad relationship in real life). If the child refuses to provide a name, go ahead and suggest one for the boy or the girl. Do not encourage children to name the illustration character after themselves. Using their own names would turn into an exposure exercise, and they have not yet learned the relaxation exercises to deal with the negative emotions that might be aroused.

The illustrations often work best if presented as a story: "This is a story about Jimmy. He was crossing the street one day and got hit by a car. Now, every time he plays by the street and a car whizzes by fast, he gets scared and thinks about the time he got hit. . . ." We've found that three of the reexperiencing items work well enough to educate the children about PTSD symptoms at their developmental level of understanding. More than three illustrations tends to make the task longer than the durations of normal attention spans for this age group:

1. Psychological distress from reminders.
2. Intrusive recollections of the event.
3. Nightmares.

As you go through this story, pick three or four points in it to ask the child if he or she makes a connection to him- or herself. "That may be like what happened/happens to you, huh?" We don't want this to become a discussion about the child, but we do want the child to make the connection that we really are talking about the child's situation indirectly with these illustrations. A simple affirmation from the child is sufficient to confirm that connection.

For children who have experienced more than one type of traumatic event, it appears OK to mention these as you talk about the illustrations—for example, "That may be like what happened to you when you were in the flood or saw that shooting."

If the child is not responding much, encourage the mother to use her influence to encourage the child to talk. Due to the nature of some traumatic events and the parent–child relationship dynamics that have developed, some children may feel that they need permission from their mother to discuss the event(s). If this issue is truly salient, it will probably be obvious to you. You could say to the mother, "Hmm. I wonder if he [she] needs a little permission from you that it's OK to talk about this stuff. What do you think?"

On rare occasions the explanation of PTSD symptoms and the illustrations work better with the child if the mother is out of the room. If you see that the child is not engaging with the illustrations, consider excusing the mom to the next room to watch on TV and try again alone with the child.

If the illustrations are too abstract and don't work well, another option to try is to use toy props to simulate the traumatic event. This is only to be done if the illustrations seem too abstract for the child's developmental level. Props should not be used to get the child to talk more about the story. It is contraindicated to reexpose the child to the memories of the event in too much detail before he or she has learned the relaxation exercises needed to deal with the anxiety.

Conclude the illustration story with a happy ending: "The boy [girl] came here and got better." Show the illustration of a child smiling. This also serves the purpose of educating the child about why he or she is coming to your office.

Finally, ask explicitly, "Do you want to come here to make your scary thoughts go away?" If the answer is affirmative, you and the child are essentially making a deal. If not, don't push it.

Example of a Story with the Illustrations: Andrew

In this example, when Andrew appears to identify with the character because they both have headaches, the therapist knows that the illustrations have clearly been successful. Andrew understands that he has new problems caused by the storm and that these problems have names.

THERAPIST: This is a story about a little boy. (*Shows the first picture of boy standing.*) What's that boy's name? You can give him a name.

ANDREW: I don't know.

THERAPIST: OK . . . let's call him . . .

ANDREW: Arthur.

THERAPIST: OK, this is a story about a little boy named Arthur. And do you know what happened to Arthur?

ANDREW: A storm came.

THERAPIST: A storm came and the water came in. And he got real, real scared. And then the storm went away but he still felt bad. Arthur felt really bad because the storm came. (*Shows a picture of a boy sitting in class, looking bored.*) In class, what's Arthur doing? Nothing. Arthur doesn't feel like doing anything since that storm came. (*Shows a picture of a boy in bed having a nightmare.*) And at night, what's he doing?

ANDREW: Lying down. He's scared.

THERAPIST: At night, he is scared and he is having nightmares. Ever since that storm came, he can't sleep at night. He is scared of the dark. And he doesn't want to leave his mom. His mom says, "I have to go," and he says, "No. No. No. Come back! Don't leave me; don't ever go away from me again!" Because they had to go away from each other during the storm, and he just wants to be with his mom. (*pause*) (*Shows a picture of a boy being angry with a peer.*) Ever since the storm, he's been getting mad. He just doesn't feel good. Do you know why, Andrew? Arthur just feels really bad ever since the storm.

ANDREW: His head hurts.

THERAPIST: Oooh. His head hurts so badly. Sometimes he has really bad headaches and his stomach hurts sometimes too.

ANDREW: The way my head aches. Like his.

THERAPIST: Like yours?

ANDREW: Yeah.

THERAPIST: (*Shows a picture of a boy smiling.*) Once he came here, Arthur started to feel better because Arthur started to talk. And I hope that you can be like Arthur, OK?

ANDREW: OK . . . I look like him. I look like him.

MOM: You look like him.

THERAPIST: You do look like him. You and Arthur have a lot of the same things going on, huh?

ANDREW: Yeah.

Give the child a snack if he or she desires one.

The Roadway Book

Show the child the three-prong binder. Explain that over the course of your meetings, this book will be filled with projects, and eventually it will be like a story of the child's life with a beginning, middle, and an end. Write the child's first name on the cover and tell him or her to *decorate the cover* with stickers and/or markers. Do not have more stickers out than you are willing to allow the child to stick on the cover. A control battle over stickers on the first day is not a good start. Each child is asked to give his or her book a name. Inappropriate name choices ought to be vetoed or investigated further, as appropriate. If a child cannot think of a name, call it the Roadway Book. You or the child then writes the new name on the cover.

Complete the first assignment for the book, Child Worksheet 1.1: About You. Help the child fill in the blanks. When asked what "the scary thing that happened to me was," some children will hesitate because they either don't want to talk about their trauma yet or they really don't know what you're talking about. Go ahead and answer quickly for the child if he or she hesitates. The point of this is to very briefly make it clear to the child why he or she is here, not to make it a quiz or a reexposure episode. In other words, you don't want to spend a lot of time talking about the traumatic event yet. That is saved for Session 5, after the child has learned relaxation exercises. Place the completed sheet in the book.

Preview the Next Session

Compliment the child's work. Tell the child that next time he or she will learn some new tools to make "scary thoughts go away."

Homework

None.

Motivation/Compliance

In addition to the above work, introduce the topic of resistance to coming back for subsequent sessions. Explain that you know from experience that parents are often reluctant to return. Sometimes it's because parents don't want to think about the trauma any more. Sometimes it's because parents don't want to expose their young children to the trauma memories any more. Sometimes it's because old memories get stirred up from parents' pasts. Explain that this is very likely to happen as the time approaches to come for the next visit. Experiencing resistance is natural and happens to almost every parent. This explanation validates the parent's experience as normal. Explain that, unfortunately, the success of the therapy depends on being able to tolerate this short-term discomfort. Finally, explain that this reluctance will lessen as the therapy proceeds and that you will be asking the parent about the presence or absence of reluctant at every session. In addition, briefly note that the child also may become resistant to returning to therapy as the work gets harder, and that you will address that issue more later.

Example of Discussing Reluctance: Andrew

The comments in the following dialogue are directed at Andrew's mother. In this example, Andrew's mother indicates that she does not really anticipate any reluctance on her part. It is important to give this warning about reluctance nevertheless because caregivers cannot really anticipate what is going to happen five or six sessions from now.

THERAPIST: There are 12 sessions. For different reasons, either the mother or the child starts to get resistant and doesn't want to come for therapy again. It could be because you have other things going on in your life. It could be because sometimes parents feel like their child is getting worse. Sometimes there may be a time when it feels like things are getting worse, but once we get through that tough spot, we get to the other side.

MOM: He needs this. There are times when Andrew just gets . . . (*Trails off in frustration.*)

THERAPIST: This reluctance of not wanting to come to the appointment is normal. That's why I am talking to you about it because it happens a lot. At some point in Sessions 1–12, he is going to say, "I don't want to talk about this any more," or you're going to feel like not going any more. So every session I'll talk to you about that. With therapy and with time, that reluctance will start to decrease.

MOM: I'm really trying to get him ready for school because he is 4 and he still has some issues. That's why we want him to come here: to try to get him ready for school.

Oppositional Defiance

✓ *Identify oppositional defiant targets.*

✓ *Address parent's leniency due to guilt.*

✓ *Make discipline plan for home.*

✓ *Make plans for grieving, if appropriate.*

✓ *Address reluctance.*

About This Session

Oppositional defiance is common in preschool children following trauma. This has been demonstrated in research and, in our experience, is the single most common reason parents bring their young children for treatment (as opposed to PTSD symptoms). Therefore, a special session is devoted to this problem at the beginning and followed up in subsequent sessions. Grieving can also be a problem with which parents need help for their young children. The appropriate parts of this session can be "pulled out" and tailored to each child. If neither defiance nor grief is a problematic issue for a child, skip this session and go on to Session 3.

The therapist spends the entire session with the child and parent together.

Materials

- Copies of relevant worksheets.

Conducting the Session

Parent and Child Welcome

The child and parent are seen together. As usual, offer a piece of candy to the child.

Review the Last Session

Begin with the usual protocol of reviewing what has been learned so far. Last week they learned about PTSD ("scary thoughts") and started the Roadway Book.

Defiance

Explain defiance. Review the initial assessment to determine how much of a problem the parent considered this issue. Reevaluate the situation now. Reconfirm the time course of defiance as a problem that either started completely new or became markedly worse after the trauma.

Example of Reviewing Defiant Behaviors: Shantice

Shantice is a 5-year-old girl who was trapped in the floodwaters of Hurricane Katrina with her grandmother and siblings when she was 4 years old. The comments in this example are directed at both the caregiver (Shantice's grandmother, Tammi) and the child in a back-and-forth manner.

THERAPIST: Defiance is when people don't do what they're grandma tells them to do, or maybe they argue or yell and that kind of thing. So, what kinds of behaviors are going on at home in terms of that?

GRANDMA: (*turning toward Shantice*) What do you do when Granny tells you to do something?

SHANTICE: Say "no."

THERAPIST: And what happens after that?

SHANTICE: They put me in time-out.

THERAPIST: Tammi, what's happening at home—when did that start?

TAMMI: She's been saying "no" since she was, like, 3. She wants to do what she wants to do, but she's been getting worse about it.

THERAPIST: When did it get worse?

TAMMI: I'd say since after the storm it's been getting worse.

Rather than ask for parents' best guesses about why this defiance developed or what to do about it, explain the theory about parental guilt and the resulting leniency with discipline. This is such a common scenario that jumping ahead in this way saves time. If this theory is wrong, the parent will tell you. Ask for opinions from the both the child and parent about whether this link between guilt and leniency is accurate. (Don't forget to ask about Dad, grandparents, or any other daily caregiver.) If confirmed, move on to the intervention.

The key is to negotiate an agreement with the mother that she will work toward ignoring her guilt or empathy for her child and enforce discipline. Explain that this approach involves a well-known cognitive therapy technique of recognizing maladaptive thoughts and replacing them with more appropriate thoughts. Instead of thinking, "Poor thing—he's been through too much already," replace it with, "Poor thing. But he still has to follow the rules. Following the rules isn't going to kill him." Parent Handout 2.1: Changing My Thoughts is an optional tool to help the parent create a discipline plan on paper.

Example of Talking to Caregivers about Guilt and Leniency: Shantice

THERAPIST: A lot of times these behaviors do get worse after traumatic events, like hurricanes and that kind of thing. And sometimes the reason for that is because parents feel that the child has been through so much already that they become more lenient with discipline. Parents become a little more lenient because when the child does something wrong, they say things to themselves like "Well, she does need to go to time-out, but she's been through so much already that I'll let this go, this one time." Has that been going on?

TAMMI: Yes, when we first evacuated, we kind of let things slide.

THERAPIST: That's really common.

TAMMI: Then, I guess, I'm just trying to get back into it now.

THERAPIST: What's the thought that goes through your head that makes you not discipline her when you normally would have before?

TAMMI: Like I said, I just think she's been going through so much, and we've had so many changes and everything. I just let it pass.

THERAPIST: Well, what helps with this a lot of the time is recognizing that guilty thought. That's the first step. The second step is to replace that guilty thought with a thought that's more appropriate and that will help you discipline her—for example, "Yes, she has been through a lot, but she still needs to know her limits." Or, "She still needs to learn the difference between right and wrong."

If parental guilt leading to leniency is not the issue, ask more questions to explore for other etiologies. Sometimes the problematic issue is the other parent or a grandparent who undermines the mother. Ask systematically how other caregivers handle discipline with the children. Remain open to all possible etiologies of defiant behavior. Another plausible scenario is a parent who needs coaching to provide more positive parental attention and tips on how to promote more prosocial behavior. That is, work on rewards for positive behavior before considering punishments for negative behavior. If no clear cause can be found, the parent management techniques reviewed in this session may still be helpful.

Next, make a list of defiant behaviors on Parent Handout 2.2: Behaviors to Change for the Roadway Book. There are usually one or two recurring situations that mothers would most like to see changed. Pick one behavior as the target behavior for the discipline plan, then narrow this behavior down to an observable, measurable unit that you (and more importantly, the mother) can tell when it has been accomplished. Review the parents' histories of discipline techniques, including use of time-out. Go over the rewards that will be used. We never select negative consequences for a discipline plan, but it is nonetheless helpful to review parents' histories to preemptively discuss, in some cases, how *not* to use negative consequences for the plan.

Write out the plan clearly and neatly on Parent Handout 2.3: Discipline Plan for Defiant Behaviors for parents to take home. It is extremely important that they leave the session with the plan written on paper. *Do not leave this planning of the task up to them to do at home.*

The child is in the room during this time and may spontaneously interject comments or can be asked for suggestions. Most importantly, the child can often be helpful in suggesting salient rewards. Sometimes the child can offer helpful information about why he or she acts up. Surprisingly, children can also sometimes admit quite openly that they know that their moms won't punish them anymore. In addition, it is clinically useful for children to hear that the therapist is backing up the mom to crack down on misbehaviors. This implicit "show of force" helps children understand that the old situation is changing.

Sometimes conflicts occur between caregivers and children during these sessions. Caregivers may use strong language, such as saying, "I hate that" about children's behavior, causing the children to react and become upset. Other times, caregivers may try to punish children in the office. Therapists need to firmly step in and lead by example when these things happen. For example, if a caregiver uses harsh language that upsets a child, the therapist can say, "Talking about it that way seems to make him [her] upset. Let's soften it a bit and say that the behavior is one you would like to see changed." If a caregiver tries to punish the child in the office, the therapist can say in a straightforward way, "I don't want the office to be a place where your child gets punished. That does bring up a good topic of what kinds of punishment to use at home."

The use of time-out as punishment at home is worth a special mention, as this use appears to be widely misunderstood. As discussed in Part I, therapists should offer advice and/or restrictions on the use of time-out to every caregiver. In addition, therapists ought to feel free to talk with caregivers about implementing a similar discipline plan for a sibling who also shows defiant behavior.

Grief

If a loved one was lost in the trauma, use this time to discuss how this loss has affected both the child and the parent. Explain the normal grieving process, and that, on average, this takes 2 years. Ask the child if he or she cries and hides it from Mom. Ask the mother if she cries and hides it from her child. Ask if it is allowed in the home to talk about the deceased. Ask if the child went to the funeral and if he or she is allowed to visit the gravesite. What does the child understand about death? Does the child persistently ask where the deceased has gone? How has the parent answered this question? Did that answer satisfy the child? The concept of "heaven" is often too abstract for very young children. A more concrete and satisfactory answer of where the deceased has gone is in a box, in the ground, at the cemetery. While caregivers may find this shocking, young children have found this type of answer helpful in our experience. Adult caregivers typically have developed personal beliefs about death and the afterlife that young children have not yet developed. Precisely how bluntly this is phrased needs to be titrated to each individual child and negotiated with the caregivers. A balance must be struck that is developmentally appropriate enough to be helpful to the children while trying to respect the beliefs about death that caregivers wish to instill in their children. Furthermore, it is helpful to remember that the reason children are asking where the deceased have gone is because their imaginations are usually worse than the truth. If children are not given an answer that they are able to comprehend, their imaginations are likely to continue to be worse than the truth.

If the child was not allowed to attend a funeral or a gravesite, or if the child simply wishes to memorialize the deceased more personally, a memorial can be created: perhaps a picture for the child's Roadway Book, a letter, a poem, or listing that person's special characteristics.

Example of Abnormal Grief: Jimmella

Abnormal grief can look a lot like depression and a lot like PTSD, and researchers and clinicians have struggled with whether or not to make traumatic grief its own disorder. The key difference seems to be that the symptoms have a connection to the lost loved one.

Jimmella was 5 years old when her father was shot and killed on a city street in a dispute over drugs. She was not present during the shooting, but she saw the crime scene and his body on the ground covered with a dark sheet. Her mother brought her for an evaluation and treatment 16 months after the loss because Jimmella was still not acting like her old self. The mother told the therapist that Jimmella asked about her daddy nearly every day: "Momma, you think Daddy is happy in heaven?" "Momma, how will I find Daddy when I go to heaven?" "I want to go see Daddy now." Her mother worried that these comments might indicate that Jimmella was suicidal. The mother also told the therapist that Jimmella had recently started saying, when she seemed to get triggered by reminders, that she should have prevented his death. After there was a schoolwide intervention several weeks ago to talk to the children about a classmate who had died, Jimmella's problems seemed to have intensified. She sat and stared at the walls, saying through her tears, "It's my fault, I think. I knew it was gonna happen." Her mother was not able to get more details from her. These behaviors differed from normal grief in that they had persisted beyond 16 months, they did not seem to be lessening (and some were getting worse), and Jimmella was distressed rather than comforted by thoughts of her father.

Give the child a snack if he or she desires one.

Prepare for the Next Session

Session 3 explores the child's feelings. This part works best if you know ahead of time what real-life *non*traumatic things have made the child scared, mad, sad, and glad. Ask the mom to give a couple examples of each, including different gradations. For example, you want an example of something that made the child a *little* mad and then something that made the child a *lot* mad.

Motivation/Compliance

Revisit the issue of any possible reluctance to come to sessions. Ask if that happened prior to today's session and, if so, to rate how strong the feeling was on a scale of 1–10. This scaling is a concrete way to determine the reduction in this reluctance as therapy proceeds. Ask what tricks were successfully used to overcome the feeling. Remember their answers so you can prompt them in the future to use the same trick. Remind parents that the reluctant feelings are short term and will get better.

Examples of tricks that caregivers have used from real cases that you might suggest include:

- Just come because the child needs it.
- Take a Xanax (short-term antianxiety medication).
- Pray.
- Come for the help so the child doesn't go through what the caregiver went through as a child without any help.
- Come for the help so the boy doesn't turn out like his father.

Ask if the child seemed reluctant as well and, if so, to rate that reluctance on a scale of 1–10. If either person was reluctant, ask for the reason(s) why to complete the Reluctance Checklist (Therapist Form 1).

Example of How to Revisit Reluctance and Rate It: Tom

Tom, a 4-year, 9-month-old boy, was a passenger in a car accident 3 months earlier. The car was rear-ended by a truck, and he was briefly pinned in the backseat. His mother was driving. She had been involved in a motor vehicle accident when she was a young adult and had refused to drive on highways for 10 years. In Session 2, the therapist had the following conversation with the mother.

THERAPIST: It's normal to be reluctant every time you come because your anxiety is really high. But, over time, that will decrease. So we hope to see it go down, and it usually does go down. So, today, how much anxiety did you have? How reluctant were you to come today?

MOM: I wanted to come, 100%. It was just the tightness in the chest. If I hadn't taken Valium, I wouldn't have come.

THERAPIST: OK, well let's try and rate that. One is none, and 10 would be the worst imaginable anxiety.

MOM: It was a 10. I wanted him to be here. It was just a matter of getting in a car and coming here.

Homework

Follow the new discipline plan. In addition, the mother's homework, if appropriate, is to catch herself feeling guilty and try to ignore it. If Parent Handout 2.1 was filled out, remind the caregiver to use it.

Mom gets her own three-prong binder for homework. Place the discipline plan and stickers in the homework binder for the mother to take home.

Preview the Next Session

Before they leave, explain that next week you will review the discipline plan and start learning new tools to make the PTSD go away. Remind them that they'll start the routine of working in separate rooms next week.

SESSION 3

Feelings

✓ *Identify distressful feelings.*
✓ *Work with parent alone.*
✓ *Address reluctance.*

About This Session

In this session children will learn to identify their emotional and bodily (somatic) feelings in relation to trauma reminders. This is the first step in their being able to practice interventions to reduce their distress. This is also a key step in the larger goal of producing a coherent narrative of the entire traumatic experience, free of distortions. Discussion and questions are used to explore emotions. Drawing on an outline of the child's body is used to explore bodily feelings.

Materials

- Copies of relevant worksheets.
- Colored pencils or markers.
- Butcher paper or large sheet of paper.

Conducting the Session

Parent and Child Welcome

Offer the candy once, then put it away.

Review the Last Session and the Homework

Briefly talk about last session, using statements, not posed as questions to the child. It is not anticipated that the child will recall much detail, but this sets up the practice of reviewing for when it becomes more important later. If a new discipline plan was started last week, review how that went. Don't spend more than about 5 minutes together at the start of each session. You just want to get a sense of how the homework went before you start working with the child. If the adult launches into a long description the child's misbehavior in front of the child, who is probably bored and restless at this point, a negative tone is set. If needed, politely explain to the mother:

> "OK, that's exactly what I want to hear about later when we split up. I want to get started with [child's name] right now, and when you and I talk later, I'd like to hear those details."

Example of How to Review the Last Session and the Homework with Mother and Child: Lucy

Lucy is a 4-year-old girl whose family had evacuated ahead of Hurricane Katrina. She was nevertheless affected by the experience of returning to find her home severely damaged. She also had been affected by a frightening experience of a lengthy X-ray procedure to try to find the cause of severe constipation when she was 3 years of age. Her discipline plan was to not call her sister any bad names for 2 out of 7 days during the prior week.

MOM: She did really well. Thursday, she was good all day long. Then, right at the end of the day, she wasn't. And then Monday and Tuesday were . . . (*Trails off in disbelief.*)

THERAPIST: And Friday and Saturday?

MOM: Friday and Saturday, she really did great. She did very good. She was very sweet. She didn't say nasty things to her sister.

THERAPIST: That is great, Lucy. Very good. Your mom is very proud of you because we know that you can do this. So, do you think you can get four more stickers this week? Do you think you can call Macy . . . ?

LUCY: Macy.

THERAPIST: That's right. Macy, and no bad names. For one more week?

LUCY: (*Nods her head in agreement.*)

Before splitting up, briefly explain what will happen next. "We're going to split up and [child's name] and I are going to work on the first tool about identifying different feelings." Escort the mother into the next room to watch you and her child on TV.

Child Alone

Teach the Child to Identify Feelings

You need to make sure that children can accurately identify different emotional states. Have a feelings chart laid out on the table for the child to look at with you. This chart should include, at a minimum, drawings of happy, sad, mad, and scared faces. First, you must educate the child about what you're going to do, so tell the child that this is a quiz about feelings. In other words, don't just dive into the task without explaining what you're doing.

Then verbally give the child scenarios that would generate each type of emotion via a facial expression. For example, say, "I bet when you eat ice cream, you feel happy, right? Show me your happy face." If the child successfully passes that one, then do another. "I bet that when another boy pushes you, you feel mad, right? Show me your mad face." And so on for sad and scared faces. Lots of different play therapy techniques, drawings, and props (e.g., a mirror) can be used to help children identify feelings. Use your creativity.

Some children, particularly those under 5 years of age, may not be able to self-identify any feelings. Nonetheless, praise them for their efforts and move forward.

Second, you need to determine if the child can accurately rate *gradations of an emotion*. For the scary feelings score, children will have to identify not just feeling scared, but they will have to differentiate between *none, a little,* and *a lot* scared. This skill cannot be assumed to be present in preschool children like it can be assumed in older populations. You will need to test to see if the child can do this. Again, this part of the session works best if you have discussed the content with the caregiver beforehand and learned what situations make the child a little scared and a lot scared (although caregiver reports are not foolproof). This also works best if you have enough real-life examples for two different discussions. The first set of examples is used for teaching the child about rating gradations of anxiety. The second set is used as a test for the child to make sure he or she understands it. Have the scary feelings score form on the table for you and the child to look at. For teaching with the first set, you might say to the child:

> "When you have to go the bathroom alone, this makes you a little scared, right? But when that spider walked on your hand, you were a lot scared. This face is a little scared [point to the face showing a little fear], and this face is a lot scared [point to the face showing a lot of fear]."

The "fish-size" method is often sufficient to help children understand *a little* versus *a lot*. Hold your hands apart a little bit to demonstrate "a little," like a fisherman showing the size of a small fish that he or she caught. Then hold your hands apart wider to demonstrate "a lot." You could also use props such as a small stack of blocks for "a little" and a higher stack of blocks for "a lot." Then, for testing with the second set, you might say to the child:

"OK, now here's your test. When I explain something that makes you scared, you point to the face of how you feel—none, a little, or a lot scared face. When your mom pushes you too high on the swing, how do you feel? [Hopefully, the child points to the 'little scared face,' and you give praise.] When your friend turned the lights off in your room that night at your house, how scared did you feel? [Hopefully, the child points to the 'a lot scared face,' and you give praise.]"

Next, for repetition, make the scary situation into a story that includes a drawing exercise. Drawing makes it concrete (and hopefully is fun) for the young child. Don't just say, "When you see a spider, you're scared, right? OK, let's draw a spider." Instead, start out by saying, for example:

"We're going to make a drawing from a story of when you get a little bit scared. So, this is a story about you, William. One day William was playing with his army soldiers in his bedroom. He was setting up the bad-guy soldiers on the floor, and then he put some good-guy soldiers up high by the window. When he put the good-guy soldiers on the windowsill, he saw a spider crawling on the window. The spider was black. This made William scared, and he yelled, really, really loud, 'Mom! Mom! A spider. Aaaaaah!' OK, let's draw that."

While you're telling the story, draw images of it on a blank sheet of paper for an extra visual aid. Depending on the age and cooperation of the child, either the child or the therapist initiates the drawing. This ought to be about something that makes the child a lot scared, as opposed to a little scared, but each clinician can make a judgment call on what situation to use for each child. The therapist will likely have to assist the child a lot with the drawing.

Next, for repetition, tape a large sheet of butcher paper on the wall, ask the child to stand against it, and outline his or her body. Ask the child to draw on this outline of his or her body where he or she feels the mad, scared, sad, and happy feelings. Some children are shy or reluctant to have their bodies outlined on the paper. This may be a problem in particular about body space/boundary issues for maltreated children. If reluctant, make a life-size outline without the child's standing against the paper. It's more important to make this activity engaging and fun than to have children comply with every step of it. If children have a hard time figuring out where to draw on the body outline, give suggestions: for example, heart pounding, head hurts, stomach knots, lump in the throat, and fidgety. Ideally, the child will do the drawing. If reluctant, you do the drawing according to what the child tells you. You may need to make the first drawing to make the exercise clear to the child. It is OK to give suggestions for drawing representations of things such as lightning bolts, sun-rays, curlicues, etc.

Next, pull out Child Worksheet 3.1: Feelings in My Body, and have the child recreate the drawing from the sheet on the wall to put in the Roadway Book. Once children have grasped the concept of talking about feelings, try to talk about feelings in response to trauma reminders in a more abstract sense.

The Roadway Book

Place the completed sheet in the book.

Homework

The homework will be on the oppositional behavior again, if needed. Explain this briefly to the child.

Preview the Next Session

Tell them that next week they will learn more about feelings and one more tool to help with trauma reminders. Give the child a snack if he or she desires one.

Parent Alone

When meeting with the parent alone, begin by briefly reviewing the last session. If a new discipline plan was started last week, discuss how it went. If the plan was not followed, you must find out in detail why and vigorously address the issues of noncompliance. Congratulate the mother on any attempt. If it was not attempted, gently ask why it was difficult. You may be walking a thin line on being too directive. Mothers who can't implement basic discipline at this point typically have an enormous amount of resistance to the idea. You should be directive, but you can soften it with humor. Remind the mother that she is the only person who *can* do this for her child. Indeed, her child *needs her* to do it for him or her. It may be evident that a particular mother simply can't attempt this intervention at this time. Perhaps the child has not been so oppositional that the mother is at the end of her rope. This breaking point time may come later, and you can explain it to the mother this way. You can also "lay it out on the table" that maybe adding tougher discipline is not in the cards. If the mother can live with the child this way, then OK. Maybe this particular form of misbehavior won't be a major issue until the child goes to school. Ultimately, remember that you can't force the mother to do anything. If the mother is unable or unwilling to work on discipline, then drop the issue and continue with the CBT work.

The mother should be bringing her homework binder with her to sessions. Ask to see it.

Teach about Feelings

Review the feelings that were covered with the child. Ask the mother if any of this information was new or surprising. Obtain any feedback as needed from the mother about what she watched you do with the child. For example, some of the child's garbled words, idiosyncratic phrases, or body language may need to be interpreted for you by the mom.

Motivation/Compliance

Revisit the issue of reluctance to come to sessions. Ask if that happened prior to today's session. Ask the mother to rate how strong her feeling was on a scale of 1–10 and record it on a fresh copy of Therapist Form 1. Once again, remind the mother that the reluctant feelings are very likely to pop up again, maybe even worse than before for a while, but that they are short term and will get better.

Next, ask the mother to grade her child's reluctance to come today on a scale of 1–10 and record it on another copy of Therapist Form 1. If the child was reluctant, ask for the reason(s) why. Again comment that this reluctance might increase as the work gets harder, and that this is natural.

Homework

The homework will be on the discipline plan again, if needed. Adjust the target behavior, reward, or overall plan as needed. Write the plan on a blank copy of Parent Handout 2.3.

Preview the Next Session

Tell them that next week they will learn more about feelings and one more tool to help with trauma reminders.

Final note: If the child showed little cooperation with or understanding of the tasks today, the rule of thumb is not to repeat the session. Move ahead next time with Session 4. Children will get more practice with these techniques in later sessions.

Coping Skills

✓ *Ascertain scary feelings score.*

✓ *Teach relaxation exercises.*

✓ *Work with parent(s).*

✓ *Address reluctance.*

About This Session

Children and parents will learn relaxation exercises in this session. These interventions will be practiced in the session and be a homework assignment for practice in the "real world." It is important for the child to learn a relaxation exercise early on so that he or she can use it later in treatment when more distressing memories are addressed.

Materials

- Copies of relevant worksheets.
- Any props needed to teach breathing exercise (e.g., pinwheel).
- Optional: training videotape of an "actor" child demonstrating the breathing and muscle relaxation exercises.

Conducting the Session

Parent and Child Welcome

Offer the candy once, then put it away.

Review the Last Session and the Homework

Briefly review last session. If you assigned the discipline plan homework, ask them how it went. If it was not attempted, talk about why it was difficult. Try to keep this all under 5 minutes and in a fairly light and positive mood. Tell the mother that you are going to teach her child how to think of, or visualize, a calming image today. Ask the mother what words you could use with her child to help him or her understand the concept. Does the child understand the word *imaginary* yet? How about *make believe* or *pretend*? The mother may be able to suggest a phrase for you to use that the child will understand.

Escort the mom into the next room to watch the session on TV and begin working with the child alone.

Child Alone

Teach Relaxation Exercises

Explain what you are going to do before you do it. Following the "full disclosure before-hand" principle, explain that you will be teaching relaxation methods to help with scary feelings, and then you will both practice them. Explain that there are three parts—muscle relaxation, creating an imaginary "happy thought," and slow breathing—and that these will be the child's tools to make the "scary feelings" or "scary thoughts" go away.

Start with muscle relaxation, since this one tends to be accepted more easily than the others. There are many acceptable ways to teach the exercise; Therapist Form 2: The Relaxing Two-Step Exercises is provided as an optional guide. This description uses counting by 2's to make it rhythmic and concrete. We've found that it's engaging to describe it as making your muscles "tight, tight" (demonstrate by squeezing your arm muscles) and then "go loose like noodles" (shake your arms around like noodles to demonstrate). You may use your own favorite method too. The point is to try to make it fun and engaging.

Next, explain happy-place imagery. Children can learn to self-soothe by replacing scary feelings with this comforting picture when they get too scared. You can call it "happy place" or "happy thought," or you may need a different term that they understand better. A happy thought can be about some event that was fun (e.g., a party), someplace calm (e.g., the beach), someplace familiar (e.g., their mother's lap), or someplace isolated (e.g., a favorite window seat in their home). Young children do not associate thoughts of being alone as happy thoughts because they are so rarely alone at this age, and many are still concerned, to some degree, about separations. Younger children's happy thoughts tend to involve exciting events with other people. Be sure to take notes on the details that the child relates. Draw the image on Child Worksheet 4.1: Draw Your Happy Place. Have fun thinking about this happy place together for about 15–30 seconds.

If children have difficulty imagining a scene with their eyes closed, it might help to practice this next skill. Tell them to look at a poster on your wall and then close their eyes but keep that picture of the poster in their head. With their eyes closed, quiz them about what's on the poster. Do this a few times until they can tell you what's on the poster with their eyes still closed.

Next, teach them about diaphragmatic breathing; children typically show the most resistance to this exercise. Try to make it engaging by putting your hand on your stomach and pointing out how it gently rises and falls with deep breaths. Have the child imitate you in a contest. Or, make it a contest about breathing in through the nose and then out through the mouth. Show the child how to do it, using exaggerated facial expressions such as a crinkled nose and puckered mouth. Another way to make it a contest is to have the child blow hard and long on something like a pinwheel. Counting and tapping out beats can also make it rhythmic and easier to remember (e.g., "Breathe in, one, two, breathe out, one, two, three"). Or, suggest that the child lie down to make it more relaxing.

Example of Learning Breathing Exercises: Andrew

THERAPIST: This is how the exercise goes. We are going to breathe in through our nose. And we're going to hold it in for two counts. And then we are going to (*exhales*) blow out through our mouths. And we are going to do that three times. You ready? These are exercises. Ready?

ANDREW: (*Nods in agreement.*)

THERAPIST: Sit down, put your hands on your lap, and look at me. Breathe in (*Andrew inhales*) through your nose. Hold it in your belly. One, two, blow it out (*exhales*), like you're blowing out a candle. OK, again, breathe in through your nose. You are going to make your belly blow up; you're brining all that air in. Hold it in your belly. One, two, blow it out. Good job.

Show a training videotape of an "actor" child demonstrating the breathing and muscle relaxation exercises if you have one (you can make your own or find examples on the Internet).

If the child appears embarrassed, offer to let him or her turn the chair away from you, or turn your own chair around.

Teach the Scary Feelings Score

Review with the child that he or she has already learned two tools: how to identify feelings and relaxation exercises. Explain that today you will teach a third tool. Show the child the "frowny face" that has three levels on Child Worksheet 4.2: Scary Feelings Score. Give examples of mild stressors and severe stressors. Guide the child in filling in this worksheet. The child may not be willing to include the trauma on the sheet yet, but give him or her permission by saying, "You're trauma might be the number 3."

Practice by having the child access a scary thought, rate its degree of scariness on Child Worksheet 4.2, and then do a relaxation exercise with the child. The scary thought ought to be about something mildly scary from everyday experience, such as seeing a spider or falling down and getting a scratched knee that bleeds. The scary thought should *not* be about their trauma. You must take the lead and do it together. Even though the task is to think about a scary thought, this can be fun and engaging. Children understand that this is just practicing in a safe office, but perhaps more importantly, by having some fun, it creates an atmosphere for the children that talking about serious topics does not have to be tense and dreadful.

Optional: Alliance Building/Playtime

If you find that you have extra time, consider just playing with the child to increase the therapeutic alliance.

Homework

Show the child the homework sheet. Tentatively select a specific target for the child, not related to the trauma, which will make him or her slightly nervous. Common examples include seeing a spider or other animals, and being in a room in the dark. Confirm later in the session with the mother before writing it down.

Preview the Next Session

Explain that next week you'll do another part of the Roadway Book and the child will learn some new things about how to control responses to trauma reminders. Offer a snack to the child, if desired.

Parent Alone

Review the Last Session and the Homework

Meeting with the caregiver alone, briefly review the last session. Look over the discipline plan homework sheet and discuss with the mother how things went during the past week. Ceremoniously place the completed homework sheet in the Roadway Book. If the homework was not completed, ask why, and help problem-solve on how future homework can be facilitated.

Teach Relaxation

Go through the steps of explaining the relaxation exercises. Make sure the mother understood what she viewed on TV. The mother will be expected to prompt the child to practice the exercises at home, so she needs to fully understand what is involved.

Some mothers may decide to use these exercises for themselves. Although this manual does not prescribe that mothers use these exercises for themselves, it is entirely acceptable to go down that path with caregivers if it seems compelling.

In addition, ask the mother how she comforts her child at home. These tried-and-true methods may be able to be worked into the relaxation exercises.

Teach the Scary Feelings Score

Review the scary feelings score on Child Worksheet 4.2. This can probably be done in abbreviated fashion if the mother was paying attention earlier. Ask the mother if any of the conversation with the child surprised her. The mother will be asked to help the child practice rating his or her scary feelings at home once next week, so the mother will need to completely understand how it works.

Have Mom Draw a Bird's-Eye-View Diagram of the Traumatic Scene

In the next session (Session 5), you will be asking the child to tell the story of his or her worst traumatic experience. It will be enormously helpful to you to already possess a map drawn of the physical layout of the scene. Ask the mom to draw a bird's-eye-view diagram of the scene on a piece of paper.

Possible Boundary Issues

By now, you will probably know if a caregiver is inappropriately intrusive beyond her child's personal boundaries for privacy and confidentiality. But even if the caregiver does not appear to have a boundary issue, it is worthwhile to give all caregivers the following spiel to preempt an awkward scene in the future:

> "In our experience, some children get embarrassed if their therapy is talked about with other family members. And if this happens, they won't do the homework or they won't talk to me anymore in therapy sessions. I just need to warn you about that ahead of time."

Motivation/Compliance

Revisit the issue of reluctance to come to sessions. Ask if that happened prior to today's session. Ask the mother to rate how strong her reluctance was on a scale of 1–10 and record it on a fresh copy of Therapist Form 1. Compare this score to the one from last week. Ask what tricks the mother successfully used to overcome the feeling. You may need to prompt the mother to use the trick she used before that worked. Once again, remind her that the reluctant feelings are very likely to pop up again, maybe even worse than before for a while, but that they are short term and will get better.

Next, ask the mother to rate the child's reluctance to come today on a scale of 1–10. If the child was reluctant, ask for the reason(s) why. Remind the mother that if reluctance is going to increase, it typically happens around Sessions 4–8 and is natural. Give the mother verbal support to encourage her to tolerate the reluctance in order to get through this hard part of the treatment.

Parent and Child Together

Homework: Test-Drive the Rating and Exercises

Fill out Parent Handout 4.1: Homework: How Much I'm Scared. Place the new relaxation homework check sheet and stickers in the homework binder. Explain that the mother will need to prompt her child to (1) expose him- or herself *one time* to a specific thing that is known to make the child slightly nervous (e.g., exposed to a spider or other animals, or being in a room in the dark), (2) rate him- or herself on Child Worksheet 4.2, and then (3) practice the relaxation exercises.

This must be done one time at home with the parent. The plan must be very explicit with the *very specific* target, date, and time written down on paper *before the mother and child leave the session*.

Explain to the mother that another purpose of this homework is to figure out which of the three relaxation exercises the child likes the best. Tell the mother to remind the child of all three exercises during the homework, but the child does not have to do all three.

Explain that the purpose of this homework is a test to see if the child really understands how to use what has been learned about these exercises. Make it enormously clear to the parent that this is to be a planned time for practicing. The mother should not make her child use the relaxation exercises in the midst of a temper tantrum. These exercises are not for that purpose.

Getting the child to do this exercise has the potential to become a battle for control. Explain to the parent extremely clearly that if the child does not want to do the exercise, he or she should never be pressured or coerced. The mother can remind the child of the reward sticker once a day, but then the matter should be dropped. The parent could enact paradoxical "Tom Sawyer" trick by doing the relaxation exercise and acting like it is enormous fun.

Keep an eye out for the subset of children who have anxiety sensitivity (Weems et al., 2007) (described in Chapter 1). That is, they get anxious about becoming anxious. These children will get so worked up about the prospect of doing any exposures that might make them anxious that they can't ever get to the point of actually doing the exposures. If you suspect this issue is present, investigate it systematically as soon as possible by interviewing the mother to confirm or disconfirm it from past history. If anxiety sensitivity appears to interfere, then candidly ask the child about this response, and the extreme sensitivity can then become an early target for homework.

Caution: Do not give caregivers permission to do this homework more than one time in the next week. There is a subset of caregivers who will either misunderstand this homework or deliberately do it differently no matter how persuasively you explain it. The worst-case scenario is a caregiver who jumps the gun and decides to start breaking her child of a phobia. For example, one caregiver decided to try to cure her child of being afraid of the dark immediately by placing her child in a dark room and telling the child to use the exercises daily. This tactic was inappropriate, too fast, too scary, and had the potential to sabotage the rest of treatment. Another caution is that if children do the exercises incorrectly for some reason, you don't want them doing that daily. There is absolutely no reason to assign this homework more than once per week.

Think of this homework as the test drive. You don't need to test drive daily. Once per week is all that is needed to practice this exercise.

Discipline Plan

If the caregiver desires to do another discipline plan, create the next plan on a blank copy of Parent Handout 2.3.

Preview the Next Session

Explain that next week you'll start talking more about the child's actual symptoms and how to use the tools he or she has learned.

Final note: If the child showed little cooperation with or understanding of the tasks today, the rule of thumb is not to repeat the session. Move ahead next time with Session 5. Children will get more practice with these exercises in later sessions.

Tell the Story

✓ Tell the story.
✓ Create the stimulus hierarchy.
✓ Explore caregiver's own trauma history and current symptoms.
✓ Address reluctance.

About This Session

Now that the child has learned about PTSD and developed tools to deal with distressing reminders, the next task is to start constructing the coherent narrative. The child will be asked to tell the whole story of what happened from start to finish. The two goals at this point are to use this session as narrative exposure for habituation to anxiety, and to build a stimulus hierarchy of distressing reminders. These topics may seem too stressful to the inexperienced clinician, but be assured that most children welcome the opportunity to talk about what happened to them.

Materials

- Copies of relevant worksheets.

Conducting the Session

Parent and Child Welcome

Offer the candy once, then put it away.

Review the Last Session and the Homework

Briefly review the last session and ask about how the homework practice went. Congratulate the child on good reports.

As usual, try to keep this review portion under 5 minutes and light and positive in mood. Escort the mom to the next room and have her watch the session on TV as you begin working with the child alone.

Child Alone

Rehearse the Relaxation Exercises

Briefly review the three relaxation tools—muscle relaxation, happy-place imagery, and diaphragmatic breathing—for practice. Repeat what you did in Session 3; at this point, you should be able to go through it much faster. Children really need to demonstrate these relaxation exercises in front of you to confirm for you that they remember how to do them.

Tell the Trauma Story

The way this task is explained to each child will depend on his or her developmental levels in verbal and abstract capacities. Basically, you need to get a complete picture of the trauma story. Explain that you're going to do something new together, why you're doing it, and that you will be taking some notes (do so on Child Worksheet 5.1: The Whole Story about What Happened). Add that you know it probably will not be fun to talk about but what happened, but that it is an important job. Older children may be able to grasp that the purpose is to develop a complete story of the trauma in order to help with their treatment. Younger children may not find their treatment to be a compelling rationale. Greater cooperation may be obtained from younger children by telling them that you need to get the whole story of the trauma for the Roadway Book. Show them the worksheet that needs to be filled in, with your help. Other explanations could be that you need the child's help to make sure you're not missing any important details of what happened, or both of you are needed as detectives who are on the lookout for clues to those scary feelings. The more competitive/oppositional children may experience increased motivation if this exercise is made into a contest.

Whereas treatments for older youth prescribe drawing exercises only part of the time and/or as needed for reluctant children, nearly all of the main office work in the PPT manual involves drawing. Drawing is a common technique with which to help younger children access past memories, express internalized thoughts and feelings (Gross & Haynes, 1998), and, in particular, describe painful traumatic memories (Malchiodi, 1997; Steele, 2012).

During the process, ask children how they felt during key parts of the trauma. Help them with cues by asking about fear, helplessness, and anger. Use their answers to these details to complete the worksheet for this session.

Young children do not have the skills yet to give lengthy, detailed narratives of past events. Without guidance, most children would tell their stories in less than a minute. After allowing each child to tell his or her story uninterrupted, you will need to go back and lead the child through the story step by step. For example:

- What was happening before the trauma occurred?
- Who was present and what were they doing?
- Were any pets affected by the trauma?
- Where exactly was everybody and what were they doing?
- What exactly was the child doing before the trauma happened?
- What were the first signs of danger?
- What was the child's first reactions?
- What did the child wish he or she had done but didn't?
- Does the child remember what he or she was wearing?
- Were any smells or tastes associated with the events?
- For car accidents: Was the other vehicle a car, van, SUV, pickup, or truck? What color was it?
- For domestic violence and maltreatment: What other objects or furniture in the environment was memorable?

Helpful comments from the therapist ought to be geared toward helping the child understand that it is important to have an organized and accurate story of what happened, including his or her thoughts and feelings along the way. Ask about smells, sights, sounds, tastes, or touch sensations that were relevant. This level of sensate detail will help the child think, feel, and behave in ways that are consistent with his or her past experience, rather than in ways that reflect a perception of the whole world as threatening and dangerous.

Take notes for yourself of a tentative stimulus hierarchy of the most distressing moments. Try to get at least five moments on the list.

Example of a Child Telling the Story: Andrew

THERAPIST: I want you to tell me everything that happened during the hurricane. I'm going to write it down. Where were you when it happened?

ANDREW: We were in the boat. (*Appears to be done with his story.*)

THERAPIST: What happened before you got in the boat?

ANDREW: They paddled. My papa and mama paddled.

THERAPIST: Who put you in the boat?

ANDREW: My mama. We were going bye-bye.

THERAPIST: Tell me what happened when the water came.

ANDREW: It was in my house. The water took it. Then I got a brand new one.

The discussion continued in this manner for another 10 minutes.

After recounting the whole story, check the anxiety level of the child. Practice the relaxation exercises regardless of the score. So, even if the child rates his or her anxiety at a 2 or 3 on the scary feelings score (Child Worksheet 4.2), still have the child use the exercises to bring down the anxiety to 1. Keep working with the child until the anxiety decreases.

Congratulate the child on his or her bravery and a job well done and ceremoniously place the worksheet in the book.

Complete the Stimulus Hierarchy

Show the child Child Worksheet 5.2: Stimulus Hierarchy, which needs to be completed in this session. Explain that the job now is to list the scary moments from the least scary to the scariest. This worksheet will be placed in the Roadway Book and used in later sessions. It's quite important that the reminders are listed in the correct order according to the degree of fear they incite. Use the notes you made earlier to rank the reminders using the scary feelings scoring. Complete Child Worksheet 5.2. Three to five items for the list are the most that young children can be expected to comprehend. Again, compliment the child on his or her bravery.

What if the child rates all reminders the same? We've found that some children rate everything as the scariest. One possible solution is to ask the caregiver to decide which are really the least scary and which are the scariest. Also keep in mind which stimuli can be turned into homework exposures and which might be physically impossible (e.g., the location of the car accident that traumatized the child is in another state). Examples of exposures that were guided by stimulus hierarchies from real cases are provided at the end of this session.

Homework

Show the child Parent Handout 5.1: Homework Check Sheet for the next week of homework (it is similar to or the same as the check sheet used the preceding week). The assignment is one exposure practice.

Preview the Next Session

Tell the child that you look forward to seeing him or her next week and offer a snack to the child as usual.

Parent Alone

The Trauma Story from the Mother's Perspective

Typically, a parent has never heard his or her child tell the whole story of the trauma from start to finish. This can be a powerful experience, not only because of the parent's feelings of empathy for the child but also in response to the memories that are stirred up in him- or herself. A good opening question is, "What did you think while you were listening to that?"

A question has been asked before by trainees of why not ask, "What did you think while you were listening to [child's name] describe the trauma?" instead of, "What did you think of while you were listening to that?" I prefer "that" for a couple of reasons. The discussions of the traumatic events are so salient when you are there in person that the word "that" conveys that the therapist "gets it," and that it need not be made so explicit in a somewhat patronizing fashion. Also, if caregivers do not, or act like they do not, understand the word "that" then that can lead to interesting clinical information.

The caregiver's responses will most likely relate to the trauma, but they can also be from her childhood experiences. The mother ought to be given the opportunity to express any and all of these. Some mothers will need no prompting to talk. Others will need an invitation to accept that it is OK to focus on themselves.

Some mothers may be visibly upset. This can be a good time to ask the mother whether her distress is evident to the child at home and possibly affecting the child. Is the kind of distress she is showing here occurring at home and can the child tell when this happens? Does the mother's distress stop her from talking about the child's trauma?

Begin thinking to yourself whether the mother is focused primarily on her child's traumatic experiences or is preoccupied by her own. The goal of this therapy is to have the mother focused on the child. If the mother appears preoccupied with other experiences, the therapist should be keeping mental or written notes about it, but this is not yet the time to be directive with her.

Example of the Caregiver's Perspective: Lucy's Mom

THERAPIST: So, tell me what you thought about that.

MOM: I noticed that when you said, "We are going to start talking about the scary things," the hurricane and all that, that she started kind of (*physically demonstrates*) putting her hands on her mouth and pulling herself in. When she was talking about the hurricane, it looked like it was bothering her. But, when she said, "No, not at all," that she wasn't scared, I don't think she was associating that with talking about the hurricane. I think she meant that talking with you, she's not scared.

You may be finding that your energy is drawn more toward dealing with the mother than the child. In contrast to protocols for older children, we encourage dealing directly with the caregiver's symptomatology. You will be talking with the mothers as much as with the children.

When you have either run out of time or run out of material, transition sensitively from this topic to stay on track with the protocol.

Review the Last Session and the Homework

Review the old worksheet for the relaxation homework. Make sure they are filling out the scary feelings score correctly. Review the relaxation exercises and make sure they still understand the purposes of these.

Possible Boundary Issues

Revisit the boundary issue if you feel that your preemptive discussion in Session 4 was not enough. For example:

> "I mentioned this last session, and I want to remind you again of how important confidentiality is for children. It appears that your child does not like [fill in the blank of the situation that embarrasses the child; e.g., the caregiver asks too many questions, the caregiver tells family members the child's personal business]. I'm afraid this could get in the way of him [her] cooperating with me. So, I want you to try to catch yourself when you're about to [fill in the blank of what the caregiver does inappropriately]. When you catch yourself about to do this, try to stop yourself. When you come in next week, tell me how many times you caught yourself, OK?"

Example of Discussing Boundary Issues: Bryson

Bryson had witnessed his father physically assault his mother several times, and now lived with his mother in the maternal grandmother's house. When Bryson and his mother arrived home after Session 4, his grandmother happened to be in the kitchen. His mother announced to the grandmother that they had just returned from Bryson's therapy session and that Bryson had learned new relaxation exercises. The mother asked Bryson to show his grandmother his new relaxation exercises. Bryson was embarrassed, probably feeling that his mother had violated his privacy by telling his grandmother that he was going to the doctor every week. He refused to show his grandmother the relaxation exercises. Furthermore, he refused to do his homework the next day, and did not want to do the relaxation exercises with the therapist the next week. When the therapist met with his mother near the end of Session 5, she volunteered that Bryson probably did not want to do the exercises because she had embarrassed him in front of his grandmother. She thought he was overreacting and deflected blame from herself. The therapist reiterated the spiel:

> "That's great that you caught that. We've seen that before that some children get embarrassed if their therapy is talked about with family members. That's going to be a bit of a problem for his counseling. Let me ask you to not talk about his therapy with his grandmother again, at least not any private details and not in front of him."

Motivation/Compliance

Revisit the issue of reluctance to come to sessions. Ask if there was any reluctance prior to today's session and, if so, to rate how strong the feeling was on a scale of 1–10. Record the score on a fresh copy of Therapist Form 1. Compare this score to their rating last week. Remind the mother that especially after today's session, the reluctant feelings are very likely to pop up again, but that they are short term and will get better.

Next, ask the mother to rate the child's reluctance to come today on a scale of 1–10. If the child was reluctant, ask for the reason(s) why. Remind the mother that if reluctance is going to increase, it typically happens around Sessions 4–8 and is natural. Give the mother verbal support to encourage her to tolerate the reluctance to get through this hard part of the treatment.

Parent and Child Together

Homework

Give the mother Parent Handout 5.1 and explain that she will need to prompt her child to practice rating his or her scary feelings score and doing the relaxation exercise of choice once in the next week, just like the preceding week (i.e., *not related to the trauma*). The plan must be very explicit with the *very specific* target, date, and time written down on paper *before they leave your office*. The mother will need to place a sticker in the box at home when the practice is completed.

As with the previous homework, you may still be trying to determine which of the three relaxation exercises the child likes the best. Tell the mother to remind the child of all three exercises during the homework, but the child does not have to do all three.

Note: In this and future homework, children may spontaneously use relaxation for innovative and/or unique purposes. For example, a child may integrate a relaxation exercise into the magical destruction of a bad object on his or her own. If this happens, go with it as long as it appears to facilitate, rather than impede, the child's healing.

Discipline Plan

If defiant behaviors are going to improve with the relatively simple discipline plans that have been used, they ought to have improved by now. It would be unusual to create additional discipline plans beyond this point, but these can be continued on a case-by-case basis, as per your judgment.

Preview the Next Session

Explain that you'll start practicing narrative exposure in the next five sessions.

Final note: If this session did not produce much detail in the trauma narrative or sufficient cooperation from the child, it is tempting to want to try to repeat it, but don't. For a variety of reasons, if it didn't work smoothly in Session 5, it is unlikely to work more smoothly 1 week later. Keep moving ahead and stay on track with the protocol because the children will get more practice with narratives in the subsequent exposures.

Easy Exposure

✓ *Begin easy narrative exposure.*

✓ *Conduct safety planning.*

✓ *Follow up on caregiver's history and symptoms.*

✓ *Address reluctance.*

About This Session

The main task of this session is to practice an easy narrative exposure. Easy items that the child can already tolerate fairly well are selected first. Over the next five sessions you will work together up the list toward the "worst moment."

A new topic is introduced today: safety planning (Runyon et al., 1998). Over the next four sessions, children will learn to identify early signs of danger, how to remove themselves from dangerous situations, and how to get help. This session focuses on the identification of early danger signals and making the safety plan.

Materials

- Copies of relevant worksheets.

Conducting the Session

Parent and Child Welcome

Offer the candy once and then put it away, as usual.

Review the Last Session and the Homework

Briefly review the last session and how the homework went in under 5 minutes. Mention that you had an important session last time and that the child was very brave in talking about the whole trauma story. Telling this story was, and is still, enormously important for making PTSD symptoms go away.

Example of Reviewing the Homework: Lawrence

Lawrence is a 6-year-old boy who witnessed his father beat and threaten his mother multiple times. In the final event, his father stabbed his mother in the arm in front of the children. The homework was to go near a neighbor's large dog that is kept behind a fence and always barks at everyone who walks past.

THERAPIST: (*looking at Lawrence*) Soooo, tell me how the homework went.

MOM: Well, we improvised a bit . . .

LAWRENCE: There was a cockroach in the house, and Mom started screaming (*laughing*), and . . .

MOM: I did. Oh, Lord, it was a big one!

LAWRENCE: . . . I thought at first something scary happened, but then she said, "It's a cockroach, Lawrence!" She wanted me to come kill it (*smiling*), and it wasn't too big, but it was big, and came right at me and at first I backed up 'cause it was kind of scary.

MOM: And it hit me right in the middle there, *this* could be his homework.

THERAPIST: Oh, good thinking.

MOM: I thought about having him rate his feelings, you know, like we were supposed to, but I just wanted him to kill it.

LAWRENCE: She said, "Get it, Lawrence. Get it. Get it" (*laughing*).

MOM: You're funny. It crawled under something so that gave me a minute to think. I said, "I think Mommy is like a jumbo scared, how about you?" And he said, "Medium."

THERAPIST: Med . . .

LAWRENCE: Then I stomped it.

THERAPIST: You stomped it?

MOM: He stomped it. Yeah. Mommy was so relieved.

LAWRENCE: It was gross.

THERAPIST: Did you do your exercises?

LAWRENCE: No.

MOM: Yes you did, boy. He did. He did his breathing and then his rating went down to nothing.

THERAPIST: I guess you didn't need to go to the neighbor's dog for the homework!

Next, split up as usual and have the caregiver watch the session on TV.

Child Alone

Easy Drawing/Imaginal Exposure

Explain that the child is going to start making the scary feelings (PTSD) go away. The child is asked to select an easy item from his or her list, draw it, imagine it, and tolerate the anxiety until any fear goes down to a rating of 1. Getting this low rating for this easy task may not take long. Give some examples first, such as going to a new place, hearing thunder, or going to the doctor. The first time is the scariest, but it gets less scary the fifth time, and is not scary at all the 10th time. This is what will happen with the PTSD list.

Producing the ideas for the children's exposures often requires creativity. To help with this component, I've listed the drawing/narrative exposures in the office and the homework exposures that we've done with over a dozen actual patients for various types of traumatic events at the end of this session.

Select an example from the child's PTSD list and explain how that the scary feeling will go away with exposure in the same way. This is the first in-office exposure.

Ask the child to draw a picture of this item, labeled the "easy reminder." Give him or her Child Worksheet 6.1: Not-Too-Scary Reminder for the Roadway Book with empty space for drawing. Overall, this task ought to last several minutes, or the amount of time it takes the child to draw the picture.

Ask for the scary feelings score at the beginning for a baseline rating and then every 3–5 minutes thereafter: "How scared are you now: none, a little, or a lot?" Keep a copy of the scary feelings score in view on the table for the child to reference. It is useful to remember that in the early sessions you are probably educating the child on how to do this exercise as much as anything.

The child can use the relaxation exercise to help him or her stay with the scene until the scary feelings go away. Do the relaxation exercises even if the child claims not to be anxious for two reasons: (1) practice, and (2) more than likely, the child is anxious but won't admit it.

Record the child's scores on Therapist Form 2: Scary Feelings Score Form. If the child stops before then, or the exposure goes on longer than 5 minutes with no change, reassure the child that this is practice and that he or she will get better at it.

Example of Sexual Assault: Martin

Martin is a 6-year-old boy who was sexually assaulted by a 13-year-old stepbrother. The assault occurred at Martin's house in their living room.

THERAPIST: So, what we are going to talk about now is what happened at home in the living room. OK?

MARTIN: (*Points to thermometer.*)

THERAPIST: You're feeling a 10? OK. What can we do?

MARTIN: (*Does relaxation exercises.*)

THERAPIST: Can you tell me what happened in the living room that is scary for you to talk about?

MARTIN: (*Moves to couch, very uncomfortable.*) He [stepbrother] came into the living room with me.

THERAPIST: I just want to tell you that nothing you say will be embarrassing or make me think differently of you. I want you to know that. We are only talking about this to help you with it. I'm just playing secretary and writing it down, but this is your story. (*pause*) So he came up behind you and did he put part of his body on you?

MARTIN: Yes.

THERAPIST: Was he your friend? Did you trust him, like, were you scared when he came behind you?

MARTIN: I thought he was my friend, but I got scared when he came behind me. (*Sits on the couch with his face down, arms over his head.*)

THERAPIST: Did what he do hurt you? Where did he hurt you on your body?

MARTIN: Yes. (*Gets up and points out on a picture where he was hurt.*)

Telling the story continued in this fashion for another 5 minutes with the therapist firmly but gently asking for additional details.

Watch out for some children, particularly boys, who don't want to admit to being scared. If you suspect this is happening, change *your* wording from "How scared are you?" to "How hard was that—none, a little, or a lot?"

After drawing the sketch, ask the child to close his or her eyes and think about it for 30 seconds (imaginal exposure).

If the child has difficulty imagining a scene with eyes closed, it might help to practice this skill first. You might try the practice that was suggested in Session 4: Tell the child to look at a poster on your wall and then close his or her eyes but to keep that picture of the poster in mind. With his or her eyes closed, quiz the child about what's on the poster. Do this a few times until the child can tell you what's on the poster with his or her eyes still closed.

Place the drawing in the Roadway Book.

Safety Planning

If this session is running long, safety planning can be delayed until Session 7 or 8.

There are two steps in this safety planning part: (1) Identify danger signals and (2) compose the actual safety plan. Examples of multiple types of trauma are provided in Chapter 2.

Explain to the child that you will start something new this week that will teach him or her how to avoid trouble in the future. Explain that the first step is to identify danger signals; the child needs to know how to tell when danger is coming before it actually happens. Each example ought to be individualized to the type of interpersonal trauma a child experienced (e.g., domestic violence, physical abuse, community violence, dog attack). You know from talking to families that, for example, before dads hit moms, they act angry and mean first.

The second step is to compose the actual safety plan to address the type of trauma the child experienced. You will write the preliminary plan on Child Worksheet 6.2: My Safety Plan. The ideal elements of a safety plan for older children are to remove themselves from the danger and to call for help if someone else (e.g., their mother) is in danger. The safety plan will be different depending on the type of trauma and the developmental age of the child.

Example of Safety Planning: Lawrence

THERAPIST: How could you tell that your parents were going to fight? How would your dad look?

LAWRENCE: He looks mean.

THERAPIST: How does he act when he's mad? Does he yell?

LAWRENCE: Yes, and he curses. At my old house, sometimes he would cry.

THERAPIST: Would he bang things and make a lot of noise?

LAWRENCE: (*Nods his head "yes."*)

THERAPIST: Yes? OK, so what I want you to do is, when you see your dad acting like that now, I want you to know some things you can do to keep yourself and your family safe. What kind of things could you do?

LAWRENCE: I could try and keep my mama back.

THERAPIST: Well, your dad is pretty big and you're pretty small. So do you think you could call 9-1-1?

LAWRENCE: Yeah, press 9-1-1. Only have to dial two 1's.

THERAPIST: Do you have any neighbors or someone whose house you could go to and tell them that something bad is happening?

LAWRENCE: I've got a lot of neighbors. I feel safe at DJ's house.

THERAPIST: OK. Could you call DJ or his mama and say, "My mom is getting hurt. Could you come help me, come pick me up?"?

LAWRENCE: (*Nods "yes."*)

THERAPIST: So, maybe, next time you see that your dad is really mad, do you think you could go to a friend's house? Or call 9-1-1 if your mom is getting really hurt?

LAWRENCE: Yeah, I can do that.

THERAPIST: OK. We'll work out a plan with your mom and practice it later.

Preview the Next Session

Next, the child will move up a bit on the scary feelings score and practice a little harder imaginal exposure.

Offer a snack to the child as usual.

Parent Alone

Ask the mother, as usual, "What did you think?" Find out where the mother's mind is primarily focused during the child's portion of the session. Is it on her child? Is it on her own thoughts and feelings about the trauma? Is it about some trauma from her own childhood? Then give the mother permission and encouragement (again) to express these thoughts and feelings to you. Follow the same guidelines from the last session.

At an appropriate time, find a way to sensitively transition to review the homework. Were the check sheets completed? If so, congratulate the mother. If not, explore why not. Make sure the mother still understands the proper use and purpose of the relaxation exercise for the child.

A Note about Mothers Who Surprise Their Children with the Homework

We've found that some mothers do not follow our carefully laid plan of conducting the trauma-related homework exposure as we discussed in sessions. Instead, they surprise the children with the exposure activity. This is not necessarily a bad thing. If the surprise homework produced a moderate amount of anxiety, the child was not overwhelmed, and the child was able to use a relaxation exercise to decrease the anxiety, then it was successful. Explore with the mother her reasons for doing it this way. She probably had a good reason. If not, and/or if the surprise was overwhelming, counsel the mother to try a more transparent tactic.

If discipline homework was assigned again for defiant behavior, go over that also.

Safety Planning

Review the safety plan with the parent as you did with the child. Discuss with the mother what she believes is feasible. You keep the worksheet for now.

Safety plans were originally created with domestic violence in mind. However, we've found safety plans helpful for just about any type of trauma. They seem to be very concrete exercises that young children can appreciate.

Some tips for mothers experiencing domestic violence include emphasizing the importance of removing themselves and their children from danger at the earliest warning signals. Review their options for calling for help from nearby friends and the police. Make a card with the plan that includes trusted friends, their addresses, and phone numbers.

One More Reminder about Possible Boundary Issues

Revisit the boundary issue if you feel that your discussions in Sessions 4 and 5 were not sufficient. Consider using Parent Handout 6.1: Respecting Boundaries. You might say the following:

"I mentioned this last session, and I want to remind you again of how important confidentiality is for children. It appears that it's still an issue that your child does not like [fill in the blank with the situation that embarrasses the child, e.g., caregiver asks too many questions, caregiver tells family members the child's personal business]. So, I want to remind you again to try to catch yourself when you're about to [fill in the blank with whatever the caregiver does inappropriately]. Let's fill out this sheet as a homework for you."

Motivation/Compliance

Review, as usual, any reluctance to come to therapy. Even if no or little resistance has been detected so far, do not let up on this task. Complete a new Therapist Form 1, as usual. The lack of resistance may be a response to your preemptive discussions about it as a possibility.

Next, ask the mother to rate the child's reluctance to come for this session on a scale of 1–10. If reluctant, ask for the reason(s) why. Remind the mother that if reluctance is going to increase, it typically happens around Sessions 4–8 and is natural. Give the mother verbal support to encourage her to tolerate any reluctance in order to get through this hard part of the treatment.

Parent and Child Together

Homework

At the end of the session, explain to them both that it is time to take the next step and add real-life (*in vivo*), not imaginary, exposure. Select an item from the easy end of the stimulus hierarchy, and assign the homework of exposing the child to that situation until his or her anxiety decreases to a rating of 1. This will, of course, require caregiver participation. As with the instruction for selecting imaginal exposures, make sure the mother and child select an easy task with which to start. Practice it once in the next week. Fill out Parent Handout 6.2: Homework Check Sheet with the mother and tell her to take this home and put it in her homework folder.

Normalize for the mother that some children regress around this point in treatment because the anxiety level is increasing. Make sure she understands how to reach you by phone if needed. Briefly state that you look forward to hearing how the real-life practice went.

Selecting a Trauma Exposure Homework: Martin

THERAPIST: The homework this week will be the first time Martin gets exposed to a real reminder of the trauma. We want to start slow and pick some kind of reminder that is not too scary. Here's the list of reminders that we've made. (*Shows the stimulus hierarchy.*)

MOM: Uh-huh.

THERAPIST: We were talking about it earlier and think that driving to the house where it happened, but not getting out of the car, would be a good start.

MOM: Driving to the old house? (*Sounds skeptical.*)

THERAPIST: Uh-huh. But you don't need to get out. Just park a couple of houses away and sit in the car for about 30 seconds.

MOM: Can you do that, Martin?

MARTIN: No, I mean, I don't know. Maybe.

MOM: (*Sighs.*) I don't know if I can go back there. (*Chuckles.*)

THERAPIST: Yeah.

MARTIN: We got our exercises, Mom.

THERAPIST: That's right. Just like we do them here. When you first get there, sit there for just about 30 seconds. Then ask Martin to rate his scary feeling score and do his exercises. Get another score after the exercises to see if it went down.

MOM: Yeah?

MARTIN: (*Shrugs.*)

THERAPIST: I think that's a good plan. I'm writing it out on the homework sheet for you.

Preview the Next Session

In the next session the exposure will be slightly more difficult.

Medium Exposure

✓ Begin medium narrative exposure.

✓ Review safety planning.

✓ Follow up on caregiver's history and symptoms.

✓ Address reluctance.

About This Session

Sessions 7 and 8 are nearly identical to each other. The aims are to provide more narrative exposure and habituation for the child, more practice with the anxiety-reducing tools, and to move up the stimulus hierarchy list. The safety plan is reviewed and rehearsed in session with puppets first and then with the child.

Materials

- Copies of relevant worksheets.

Conducting the Session

Parent and Child Welcome

Offer the candy and then put it away, as usual.

Review the Last Session and the Homework

Review, in less than 5 minutes, the last session and how the homework went. Did the child practice the real-life exposure? If so, review what the child did, his or her feelings during the exposure, and how the anxiety resolved. Be sure to ask about multiple possible sensory experiences, such as sight, smell, hearing, taste, and touch.

Next, escort the mother to the other room, as usual.

Child Alone

Medium Drawing/Imaginal Exposure

Just like last week, explain that the child is going to make the "scary feelings" or "scary thoughts" go away. If the child had trouble with the easy item last time, start with that one again in this session. If not, move up to a harder item on the stimulus hierarchy. The child will need to tolerate the anxiety until his or her fear decreases to a rating of 1. You might give nontrauma examples again to educate the child on the purpose of this exercise, such as going to a new place, hearing thunder, or going to the doctor. Tell the child that the first time is the scariest, but it gets less scary by the fifth time, and is not scary at all the 10th time; this gradual lessening in fear will occur for each item on the PTSD list.

Pick a medium example from the list and explain how that the scary feeling will go away with exposure. Get the baseline scary feelings score and write it on Therapist Form 2.

Finally, have the child draw a picture of this item. Use Child Worksheet 7.1: Medium-Scary Reminder, with empty space for drawing. Tell the child to stay in the situation until he or she is not scared at all—and may even get bored. The child can use the relaxation exercise to help him or her stay with the scene until the scary feelings go away.

Ask for the scary feelings score every 3–5 minutes (or whatever pace seems appropriate for each child), and record each score on Therapist Form 2. Keep a copy of the scary feelings score in view on the table. Do the relaxation exercises. When the scary feelings score has gone down to 1, you can stop. If the child stops before then, or the exposure goes on longer than 5 minutes with no change, reassure the child that this is practice and that he or she will get better at it.

Example of Being Assertive with the Pace of Exposures: Lawrence

THERAPIST: Are you having jumbo scared feelings, extra-large, large, medium, or small scared feelings?

LAWRENCE: Extra-large.

THERAPIST: So this is a thermometer about sad feelings. How many sad feelings are you having right now?

LAWRENCE: (No answer, just keeps drawing.)

THERAPIST: Do you feel like crying right now?

LAWRENCE: Yeah. I feel like I'm about to throw up.

THERAPIST: Let's stop and do some relaxation techniques, OK? Do you remember the breathing?

LAWRENCE: (Automatically starts doing the exercises.)

THERAPIST: Very good. Let's do it two more times, then we can do muscles.

LAWRENCE: (*Does three repetitions of the exercises.*)

THERAPIST: Feeling better?

LAWRENCE: Yeah.

THERAPIST: Good job. Let's try the drawing again.

After drawing the picture, ask the child to close his or her eyes and think about the event for 30 seconds (imaginal exposure). Ask for a scary feelings score at the end and use relaxation if needed to get it down to a rating of 1.

Watch out for children who don't like doing the relaxation exercises and report a lack of anxiety to get out of doing it.

Place the drawing in the Roadway Book.

Safety Planning

Review the safety plan from last week, reminding the child of the danger signals that were identified and what the child's response to those signals would be. Then use two puppets to play out the danger scenario. One puppet is the angry person, and the other puppet is the child. The therapist will need to demonstrate an angry face as one of the danger signals. In our experience, children easily grasp that the action can go back and forth between the puppets and the therapists' faces and voices. Provide a running commentary on the action to emphasize the danger signals. The child puppet recognizes the danger signals and then enacts the safety plan.

Next, use only the angry puppet and have the child role-play the child's part. The child may choose to use the child puppet or simply talk for him- or herself as the child. Display the danger signals again and ask the child to identify them and what he or she will do to enact the safety plan.

Example of Safety Planning: Child Role-Plays with Puppets: Lucy

Spot is Lucy's puppet; Dot is the therapist's puppet. It does not need to be made explicit as to whether Spot and Dot represent anyone in particular. In fact, if therapists tried to explain that Spot is the representation of the child and Dot is the representation of a therapist or mother this would add a layer of abstract cognitive thought to the exercise that is both somewhat challenging for this age group and unnecessarily complicates the exercise. Children intuitively understand that Spot and Dot do not need an introduction or an explicit relationship.

THERAPIST: Hi, Spot. I heard that you're really smart and you know what to do to stay safe from a hurricane. Is that true?

LUCY: I think.

THERAPIST: What can I do?

LUCY: I can bring my stuffed animals.

THERAPIST: OK. How will we know if a hurricane is coming?

LUCY: We can check the weather, the weather on the news. It'll tell us if rain comes and if sun comes and hurricanes. I'm a little . . . I'm a lot scared of hurricanes.

THERAPIST: Yeah, I'm scared of hurricanes too.

LUCY: But I know what to do when I'm scared of hurricanes. You do your breathing exercises.

THERAPIST: Yeah. Let's do them now.

LUCY: (*Begins breathing exercises.*)

Preview the Next Session

Next, the child will move up a bit on the scary feelings score and practice a little harder imaginal exposure from the stimulus hierarchy.

Offer a snack to the child as usual.

Parent Alone

Check in with the mother again on what she thought while watching this portion with her child. "Well, what did you think of that?" Continue to give the mother permission and encouragement to express her own thoughts and feelings to you. By now you will have settled into a rather predictable routine with the caregivers. Some caregivers have little to talk about, some have a lot to talk about; some are focused on their children, some are focused on themselves; some have no crises to deal with, some have a new crisis almost every week to address.

If it has become apparent that the mother seems preoccupied by her own past experiences, it is often best to allow her the opportunity to talk. Remember that this manual sets aside time for the therapist and caregiver to meet every session for several reasons. One reason is that it allows time for caregivers to process their new discoveries about their children in the hopes of becoming better attuned to their internal worlds. Another reason is to benefit from caregivers' ability to interpret their children's language and body language. A third is that it can be supportive therapy for the caregivers. Active listening and advice giving are valuable and supportive functions. If caregivers are telling you about their past experiences, it is probably because they feel a need to do so and can benefit from your active listening. In that sense, your job is to encourage talking and gather information. These concerns need to be balanced with the limited time you have in treatment.

At an appropriate time, find a way to sensitively transition to review the homework. Were the check sheets completed? If so, congratulate the mother. If not, explore why not. Make sure the mother still understands the proper use and purpose of the relaxation exercise for the child.

If discipline homework was assigned again for defiant behavior, go over that also.

Safety Planning

Review the child's safety plan with the parent. Make sure that the mother can identify the salient danger signals in the child's plan, which may be more subtle than the signals that her child can detect. For example, a child may sense danger when a father has a red face and is yelling, but a mother may sense the danger minutes earlier when the father walked ominously through the kitchen without speaking to her and before he started yelling. The point of this discussion is not for the child to change his/her danger signal, but to attune the mother to the concept of danger signals. By having the conversation at a different level of subtlety with the caregiver than with the child, this demonstrates competency on the part of the therapist.

Motivation/Compliance

Review, as usual, any reluctance to come to therapy. Reluctance should be decreasing. Complete a new Therapist Form 1, as usual, for both mother and child. Remind the mother that if reluctance is going to increase, it typically occurs around Sessions 4–8 and is natural. Give the mother verbal support to encourage her to tolerate the reluctance in order to get through this hard part of the treatment.

Parent and Child Together

Homework

At the end, explain that the mother and child need to jointly select another real-life (*in vivo*) exposure to practice for homework, ideally, an item from the middle part of the stimulus hierarchy. The selection of the exposure is a negotiation that also involves the therapist. The child needs to stay with the situation until the anxiety goes down to a rating of 1. This homework will, of course, require the parent's participation. Practice it once in the next week. Complete Parent Handout 7.1: Homework Check Sheet with the caregiver, who then takes it home for her homework binder.

Preview the Next Session

Briefly state that you look forward to hearing how the real-life practice went. Next week, you'll work on a little bit harder exposure.

SESSION 8

Medium Exposure

✓ *Begin medium narrative exposure.*

✓ *Review safety planning.*

✓ *Follow up on the caregiver's history and symptoms.*

✓ *Address reluctance.*

About This Session

This session is nearly identical to Session 7. You will move up the stimulus hierarchy list in practicing the narrative exposure and in selecting goals for the homework, and make progress on the safety plan.

Materials

- Copies of relevant worksheets.

Conducting the Session

Parent and Child Welcome

Offer the candy and then put it away, as usual.

Review the Last Session and the Homework

Ask how the homework went and review it in less than 5 minutes. Did the child practice the real-life exposure? If so, review what the child did, his or her feelings during the exposure, and how the anxiety resolved. Be sure to ask about multiple possible sensory experiences, such as sight, smell, hearing, taste, and touch.

Example of Review of Homework: Tom

In this example, the therapist and mother discover that the child's reaction to a trauma reminder is anger, not fear or anxiety.

THERAPIST: So, Tom, tell me how your homework went? Did you and your mom go see a black truck?

TOM: Yes, one. Then, we went and saw another one.

MOM: Yeah, when we took a walk.

THERAPIST: When you saw that black truck, how scared were you?

TOM: (*Holds up 10 fingers.*)

THERAPIST: Wow, so you were really scared. And what did you do to get not so scared?

TOM: (*Demonstrates interlacing and twisting the fingers of both hands.*)

THERAPIST: You were tightening your muscles?

MOM: We did noodles. And we did breathing . . . he was angry, very angry.

THERAPIST: Your mom says you were angry when you saw the truck. What do you do when you get angry?

TOM: I don't know.

MOM: He hits. He wanted to kick and hit the truck.

TOM: I didn't do it. We did breathing.

THERAPIST: Did that help? Did you still want to hit the truck?

TOM: (*Nods "yes."*)

MOM: But, he stopped swinging at it. He kept saying, "Bad. It's a bad truck."

THERAPIST: Remember how you went to see the stop sign and you did your exercises and then you weren't so scared anymore? If you keep going to see the black truck, and keep doing your exercises, then you won't be scared or angry any more. So, you'll keep trying it?

TOM: OK.

Next, take the mother to the other room, as usual, to watch the session on the TV monitor.

Child Alone

Medium Drawing/Imaginal Exposure

Working with the child alone, just like last week, explain that the child is going to make his or her PTSD go away. If the child had trouble with the item from last week, start with that one again in this session. If not, move up to a harder item on their stimulus hierarchy. Remember that you may need to be explicit in explaining that you are moving up to a "morescary" item this week. Some children believe that since they did a drawing last week, it's stupid to do the same thing again this week ("I already did that!"). Explain briefly how this is a new one. Follow the instructions from the last session in the protocol.

Ask the child to draw the scene on Child Worksheet 8.1: Medium-Scary Reminder. During the drawing, an optional task for the therapist is to detect any negative relational feelings the child has toward close adults because of the trauma. Ease into this area by first asking who the child believes was at fault for what happened. If needed, go through a menu of logical possibilities—for example, the driver of the other car, the perpetrator, Dad, Mom, the police. At some point, ask about the child's mother/caregiver because she is the one involved in the treatment.

Possible questions include "Do you feel mad at [name of person]?" If so, ask why. Eventually, proceed to asking whom the child blames for what happened.

The other salient persons involved in the traumas will usually have been adults, but keep in mind that you may need to ask about other children. Also, be sure to ask if the child thinks it's his or her own fault. For example:

- Is there something the child thinks he or she should have done to prevent the trauma?
- Is there something the child wishes he or she could do about it now?
- Is there something the child wishes he or she could do now to make him- or herself feel better?

You don't need to have advice or a plan to address the child's answers to these questions right now. You just need to gather data about what the child is thinking. If distorted thoughts or feelings are detected, caution is urged not to prematurely assume distortion. For example, a child may say that he or she blames Mom for the fight that led to the battering. With more careful exploration, this may lead to finding new details about the event that the mother wasn't willing to disclose at first.

If negative or ambivalent feelings are detected, it is important to express empathy and to acknowledge that the child was heard. This can be as simple as a sympathetic "Ooh," or saying, "I'm sorry that happened to you," or "That's important and we need to talk with your mom about that too."

Ask the child for a scary feelings score at baseline and every 3–5 minutes during the drawing and record them on Therapist Form 2.

Use one or more relaxation exercises for practice even if the child claims not to have any anxiety.

Have the child do the imaginal exposure next for 30 seconds with eyes closed. Recheck scary feelings score.

Safety Planning

Review the safety plan. Role-play the danger signals using the puppets again. Have the child identify the danger signals and rehearse his or her safety plan. Write out the current version of the safety plan on Child Worksheet 8.2: Safety Plan.

Preview the Next Session

Next, the child will move up a bit on the stimulus hierarchy and practice a little harder imaginal exposure.

Offer a snack to the child as usual.

Parent Alone

Almost identical to the last session, check in with the mother about what is most pressing on her mind. If you began a discussion last week about the mother's past experiences, this needs to be followed up this week. The mother has undoubtedly thought about your discussion at home over the last week. Ask for her thoughts. See if there has been any shift in her thinking. The goal this week is, again, simply to listen, think out loud about the topic with the mother, and don't give any premature directives.

If mothers seem critical or offended by anything their children brought up, remind them to be nonjudgmental for now because we're teaching children to talk about their feelings. If you asked the child about blame and you suspect the child has some distorted cognitions, ask the mother to help clarify them. This may lead to uncovering new details about the event that the mother wasn't willing to disclose at first. Make notes of distorted thoughts or feelings that may need to be addressed later.

Optionally, use this opportunity to append an inquiry about angry relational feelings, just as you did with the child. Ask the same questions you asked the child. Start with an open-ended question to ascertain how the mother feels about the other person(s). Then move to more specific questions, such as, "Do you feel mad at [name of person]?" If so, ask why. Eventually, proceed to asking whom the mother blames for what happened. Caution is urged about confronting a mother as to whether her perceptions are really distorted or not. It is natural for parents to blame themselves because they are protective of their children. Blaming themselves is not a bad thing per se. On the other hand, if the self-blame leads to leniency with discipline or personal problems, then it could be addressed later.

If the family is the type that tends to present a "crisis of the week," continue supporting the mother in her efforts to cope with the latest crisis as much as time allows.

Safety Planning

Explain that the new homework assignment is to rehearse the safety plan in the home once before the next session. The parent will need to initiate the rehearsal at home. The parent can either role-play the danger signals herself or just verbally describe them. The child will be asked to walk through the safety plan.

Motivation/Compliance

Review, as usual, any reluctance to come to therapy. Fill out a new Therapist Form 1 as usual. Assure the mother that any increased reluctance is normal as the drawing and *in vivo* exposures become more challenging for the child.

Parent and Child Together

Homework

Bring the child back into room. Explain that the caregiver and the child need to select, in negotiation with the therapist, another real-life (*in vivo*) exposure to practice for homework, ideally an item a bit further up the stimulus hierarchy from the previous selection. The child needs to stay with the situation until the anxiety goes down to a rating of 1. This homework will, of course, require the parent's participation. Practice it once in the next week. Complete Parent Handout 8.1: Homework Check Sheet and give to the caregiver to take home for her homework binder.

An additional homework this week is to rehearse the safety plan in the home, as described above. You can photocopy Child Worksheet 8.2 if the mother would like the plan on paper to remind her of the plan later. At home, the mother and child must walk through the child's safety plan. Explain that you need to see if the plan should be tweaked after they walk through it in the real environment.

Preview the Next Session

Briefly state that you look forward to hearing how the real-life practice went. Next week, you'll work on a little bit harder exposure.

Worst Exposure

✓ *Begin worst-moment narrative exposure.*

✓ *Conduct safety planning.*

✓ *Follow up on caregiver's history and symptoms.*

✓ *Address reluctance.*

About This Session

The next two sessions should focus on exposing the child to the worst moment—the highest item on the stimulus hierarchy with a scary feelings score of 3. The same format is used as in the previous three sessions. Children who have had difficulty advancing up the stimulus hierarchy should still be encouraged to focus on their worst moment in this session.

The safety plan should have been rehearsed at home over the last week.

Materials

- Copies of relevant worksheets.

Conducting the Session

Parent and Child Welcome

Offer the candy and then put it away, as usual.

Review the Last Session and the Homework

Ask how the homework went and review it in less than 5 minutes. Did the child practice the real-life exposure? Go over it as usual.

Then escort the mother to the other room, as usual.

Example of Review of Homework: Lawrence

THERAPIST: How was the last week? Did you guys do any homework?

MOM: We did. We went to the house physically. We even went to look into the house.

LAWRENCE: We went in the front yard.

MOM: We peeked through the windows because the people moved. We got to see the living room where Mama got stabbed, and they had cleaned all the blood up.

THERAPIST: So, Lawrence, when you saw all that, how were you feeling? Like what number on the stress thermometer would you think?

LAWRENCE: I was scared. (*Points to 10 on thermometer picture.*)

Child Alone

Worst-Moment Drawing/Imaginal Exposure

Just like last week, explain that the child is going to make his or her PTSD go away. If the child had trouble with the item from last week, start with that one again in this session. If not, move up to the child's worst moment. He or she will need to tolerate the anxiety until the fear goes down to a rating of 1. By now, giving examples of how this process works should not be needed.

Have the child draw the scene on Child Worksheet 9.1: Worst-Moment Reminder.

Ask for scary feelings score at baseline and every 3–5 minutes and record them on Therapist Form 2.

Use one or more relaxation exercises for practice even if child claims not to have any anxiety.

Have the child do the imaginal exposure for 30 seconds with eyes closed. Recheck the child's scary feelings score.

If the stress rating is not decreasing, make sure the child is using the relaxation exercise. If the stress does not come down to a rating of 1 after 30 minutes, you will need to intervene. Engage the child in a conversation about what he or she is thinking. Gradually shift the conversation away from the trauma reminder and distract the child with other topics. If this doesn't work, it may be appropriate to bring the mother into the room to help soothe and/or distract the child. The child can then be led to the next room and engaged with the usual snack and games. The child should not leave the office with a rating still above 1. The session may have to be prolonged.

Place the drawing in the Roadway Book.

Safety Planning

This discussion can take place without puppets, but puppets can be used if that helps.

Ask the child if he or she practiced the safety plan at home last week. If so, how did it go? In the process, review the danger signals and the safety plan for one more iteration with the child, and troubleshoot as needed. Some examples of troubleshooting may be as follows:

- A girl's safety plan for hurricanes was to pack her suitcase with a change of clothes and a couple of her favorite toys. When they practiced the safety plan at home, they discovered that they could not find her suitcase. They modified the plan by switching to a large shoulder bag that Mom loaned her.
- A boy's safety plan for domestic violence was to call his grandmother who lived down the street. When they practiced the safety plan at home, they realized that grandmother's phone number was not written down anywhere. They modified the plan by taping grandmother's phone number on the wall by the phone and on the refrigerator.
- A girl's safety plan for sexual abuse was to tell her mother as soon as she found herself left alone with any older boys or men. When they practiced the plan at home, they found that the girl thought it meant only men whom she had never met before. They modified the plan to include relatives and acquaintances that she already knew.

If the safety plan was not practiced, ask why not.

Preview the Next Session

The plan is for the child to practice the worst-moment exposure again.

Offer a snack to the child, as usual.

Parent Alone

Follow the usual procedure with the mother. If you have been discussing the mother's preoccupation with her own past experiences the last 2 weeks, now may be the time to start being directive, if needed.

Some mothers may simply need time to keep talking about their own pasts. Sometimes it is hard to tell if this is being productive or not. If it's not clear, then try this rule of thumb: As long as the mother is talking and the sessions are not lasting too long for the child to play contentedly in the next room, then keep listening up to 90 minutes for the full session.

There are 3 weeks left in the protocol. It may be time to make a joint decision about seeking a referral for the mother's individual therapy.

Before ending, be sure to review the homework. Were the check sheets completed? If so, congratulate the mother. If not, explore why not.

The child's oppositional problems ought to have decreased significantly by now if the mother has been following the homework. If the behaviors have not substantially lessened by this point (whether they need a different intervention or the mother has not followed through on the homework), further time ought not to be spent on this topic in the protocol.

Safety Planning

Ask the parent if she and her child practiced the safety plan at home last week. If they did, how did it go? In the process, review the danger signals and the safety plan for one more iteration with the parent. If the safety plan was not practiced, ask why not? Troubleshoot as needed.

Motivation/Compliance

Review, as usual, any reluctance to come to therapy. Be sure to get the rating between 1 and 10 and record it on a fresh copy of Therapist Form 1. The reluctance, whether by mother or child or both, should be decreasing.

Parent and Child Together

Homework

Bring the child back into the room and explain that caregiver and child needs to pick (with the therapist's agreement) another real-life exposure to practice for homework. The child, ideally, is able to choose a more difficult item than last week. The child needs to stay with the situation until the anxiety decreases to a rating of 1. The child should practice this exposure once in the next week, under the guidance of the parent. Complete Parent Handout 9.1: Homework Check Sheet and give to the caregiver to take home for her homework binder.

Preview the Next Session

Next week will be similar to this week. Tell them there are three more sessions left.

Worst Exposure

✓ Begin worst-moment narrative exposure.

✓ Start reviewing the Roadway Book.

✓ Follow up on caregiver's history and symptoms.

✓ Address reluctance.

About This Session

This session is nearly identical to Session 9 except that the safety planning has been completed and the review of the Roadway Book begins. The child, mother, and therapist will begin the process of reviewing the Roadway Book together. This review will be accomplished gradually over these final three sessions.

Materials

- Copies of relevant worksheets.

Conducting the Session

Parent and Child Welcome

Offer the candy and then put it away, as usual.

Review the Last Session and the Homework

Ask how the homework went and review it in less than 5 minutes. Did the child practice the real-life exposure? Briefly discuss how it went, as usual.

Child Alone

Worst-Moment Drawing/Imaginal Exposure

If the child had trouble with the item from last week, start with that one again this time. If not, move up to his or her worst moment. The child will need to tolerate the anxiety until the fear goes down to a rating of 1. By now, giving examples of how this process works should not be needed.

Have the child draw the scene on Child Worksheet 10.1: Worst-Moment Reminder.

Ask for the scary feelings score at baseline and every 3–5 minutes and record them on Therapist Form 2.

Use one or more relaxation exercises for practice, even if child claims not to have any anxiety.

Have the child do the imaginal exposure for 30 seconds with eyes closed. Recheck the child's scary feelings score.

Place the drawing in the Roadway Book.

Preview the Next Session

Talk about planning for the future.

Offer the snack to the child, as usual.

Parent Alone

Follow the usual procedure with the mother.

Before ending, be sure to review the homework. Were the check sheets completed? If so, congratulate the mother. If not, explore why not.

Follow up on the oppositional behavior plan if that is still a problem.

Motivation/Compliance

Review, as usual, any reluctance to come to therapy. Be sure to get the rating between 1 and 10 and record it on a fresh copy of Therapist Form 1. Reluctance should be decreasing.

Review of the Roadway Book

Bring the child back into the room so that the review is conducted with the child and parent together. Review the importance of every single page for Sessions 1–6. It is a tall order for a child to be in charge of this task, so you, the therapist, are in charge of exploring the pages and turning to the next one at an appropriate pace. This should take 5–15 minutes.

Example of How to Introduce and Start Review of the Roadway Book: Lucy

THERAPIST: So, today we're going to show Mommy your book, OK? Just half of it today. We're going to start at the very beginning and show her all the work you've been doing. We talked about how you're not going to say mean things to Macy. Do you remember that?

LUCY: Yes. And I would get stickers.

THERAPIST: Yeah. Look at how well you did. The first week you got three stickers and then the next week you got . . .

LUCY: Stickers everywhere!

THERAPIST: (*Flips to the next page.*) This is when you got all those stickers for doing your breathing exercises. (*Flips again.*) All of these stickers are for saying no mean things to Macy.

MOM: I remember when you started doing your breathing exercises.

LUCY: Look at all the stickers!

THERAPIST: How many days did you have to practice your breathing?

LUCY: Five days.

THERAPIST: And you did such a good job! Then we talked about the feelings in your body. What are some of those feelings?

LUCY: Happy, mad, sad, scared, afraid.

THERAPIST: Very good. Don't forget how to say if you're a little scared or a lot scared. Do you want to show this to your mom?

LUCY: (*Shows her mom a picture she drew in the book.*)

MOM: It's very nice, Lucy. Were you scared?

THERAPIST: That would be a good time to show your mom how scared you are, OK? Remember that. You can always tell her if you're scared.

Parent and Child Together

Homework

Explain that the caregiver and the child needs to choose another real-life exposure to practice for homework—ideally, a more difficult item than last week. The child needs to stay with the situation until the anxiety goes down to a rating of 1. It should be practiced once in the next week. The mother takes home the completed Parent Handout 10.1: Homework Check Sheet for her homework binder.

Preview the Next Session

Tell them there are only two more sessions left and that you need to start preparing to say goodbye. Next week you will talk about how to use their tools in the future.

Relapse Prevention

✓ *Provide information about relapse prevention.*

✓ *Review the Roadway Book.*

✓ *Make plans to terminate.*

About This Session

PTSD symptoms ought to be markedly reduced by now. You can begin to talk about the future more and what to expect. Relapse, in the sense of a return of some symptoms from time to time, is a common occurrence, and the child and parent need to anticipate this. They first need to understand that a recurrence of symptoms is natural and doesn't mean the end of the world. Then they need to be prepared to use the tools they have learned when this relapse occurs.

The review of the Roadway Book advances to cover Sessions 7–11.

Materials

• Copies of relevant worksheets.

Conducting the Session

Parent and Child Welcome

Offer the candy and then put it away, as usual. Remind the child that you have only two more sessions left.

Review the Last Session and the Homework

Ask how the homework went and review it in less than 5 minutes. Did the child practice the real-life exposure? Go over it, as usual.

Child Alone

Provide Information about Relapse Prevention

Remind the child that a lot of the bad feelings have gone away and don't bother him or her any more. Things will probably stay that way, but sometimes bad memories jump back up and scare us. Talk about this possibility in the time frame of tomorrow or next week and explain that it is normal.

First, ask the child if he or she might do something tomorrow or the next day that would bring back a bad memory. If the child has difficulty with the concept of *tomorrow*, consider showing the child a calendar to make it more concrete. If the child can't think of something, think of a salient example; Select an item from the middle of the child's stimulus hierarchy list so as not to pick the scariest moment. Tell a brief story about how the child might be somewhere next week when he or she encounters a bad reminder.

Have the child draw a picture of this situation on Child Worksheet 11.1: Near-Future Reminder. Ask the child what he or she would do. Appropriate answers would be to wait it out until he or she feels less scared, do the relaxation exercises, or talk to someone until he or she feels better.

Example of How to Draw the Near Future: Lucy

Lucy had two types of traumas: a scary X-ray procedure when she was 3 years old and Hurricane Katrina when she was 4 years old. The therapist and Lucy decided to focus on the X-ray procedure for this exercise because she would have future doctor visits.

THERAPIST: What is something that would remind you of going to the doctor?

LUCY: Bad stuff. When I have to have a shot.

THERAPIST: When do you have to go back for the doctor to put the tube in and you have to lie on the cold table?

LUCY: I don't know.

THERAPIST: Let's draw a picture of when that happens.

LUCY: (*Draws a picture of the doctor's office.*)

THERAPIST: So when you go to the doctor to have the tube put in, what can you do to not be so scared?

LUCY: Calm down. We have to do all the exercises. And more breathing exercises.

THERAPIST: And can you tell your mom how scared you are?

LUCY: Yes.

Next, ask the child to draw a picture of them when he or she is grown up. If the child has an older sibling, that may be a better age on which to focus. If the child has difficulty with concept of being *grown up*, make it more concrete by drawing a picture with a little child next to a bigger drawing of the child all grown up. Then ask the child to try to think of a situation then that might bring back a bad memory. You may have to help the child think of salient example, as above, by providing a prompt from the stimulus hierarchy. Have the child draw a picture of this situation on Child Worksheet 11.2: Distant-Future Reminder. Again, ask the child how he or she could handle the situation to make the bad feelings go away.

Talking about the long-term future is a developmental impossibility for most preschool children. They can talk about what they want to be when they grow up, but they have no sense of how far away that is in the future. The future to them is tomorrow or, at the most, next week. Concentrate on that time frame. However, make an attempt to explore longer-term planning capacities to see if an individual child is able to grasp the concept.

Place the drawings in the Roadway Book.

Example of a Distant-Future Reminder: Andrew

THERAPIST: Can you draw a picture of you as a grown-up? When you're a big man and older? OK? This should be a picture of Andrew all grown up.

ANDREW: (*Draws a picture.*)

THERAPIST: What's something that might happen that would remind you of all the scary things when you were young? What scared you when you were growing up?

ANDREW: The dark scared me.

THERAPIST: And when you're grown up and you see the dark, what can you do to make the scary feelings go away?

ANDREW: My exercises.

THERAPIST: And then would you still be scared?

ANDREW: No.

THERAPIST: Just remember that if you're scared, you can always do your exercises, even when you're old.

Ask for the scary feelings scores and record them on Therapist Form 2. The purpose of asking for these scores is solely to check on the child's level of anxiety. This is not meant to be one of the graded exposure exercises. Spend extra time for relaxation or distraction if the score is above a rating of 1.

Preview the Next Session

Tell the child that next week is the last week and you will have a graduation. Ask for ideas for a special snack for the next session. These need to be small food items (such as a cupcake or candy, not meals). (Tip: Do not call this a "party" or "ceremony." Children this age might think a party means other children, a tea party, a spacewalk, balloons, cake, etc.)

Offer a snack to the child, as usual.

Parent Alone

Make sure that the mother is aware that the next session is the last one. This reminder will help her gauge the time remaining and what topics she feels compelled to raise.

If the mother's preoccupation with her own past experiences has been a relevant topic in past sessions, make sure to review that again, as in Sessions 9 and 10.

Be sure to review the homework. Were the check sheets completed? If so, congratulate the mother. If not, explore why not.

Spend some time reviewing the child's overall progress by comparing his or her presenting symptoms to the child's and mother's current reports. Get a sense of the mother's satisfaction with treatment progress. If the mother has specific complaints, you may want to use this session and the last session to address these—whether for the first time or yet again. This is not only good "customer service" but also an acknowledgment that trauma symptoms can be many and diverse, and you may not have had time to address all of them. For example, sleep difficulty is often a difficult symptom to treat, for a variety of reasons. It is also one of the symptoms that most distresses a parent because it can cause lack of sleep for the whole family. You may not have had time to talk about sleep hygiene principles and make suggestions on how to handle this issue.

Start to tie up any loose ends with the personal issues the mother has been addressing. For example, if you ran out of time when she was telling the story of her father's domestic abuse of her mother, make sure to offer the time to finish that story for closure with you. Or, if her main concern has been a custody battle with her ex-husband, offer the time for her to discuss her concerns and help her problem-solve if appropriate.

Finally, if the mother has been symptomatic, you must make an estimate of whether she needs continued individual treatment and, if so, make referral suggestions. Make sure to follow up any referral suggestions at the last session.

Motivation/Compliance

Review any reluctance to come to this session, on a scale of 1–10, and record it on a fresh copy of Therapist Form 1. Reluctance to come to the last session should not be an issue.

Parent and Child Together

Review of the Roadway Book

Bring the child back into the room and review the Roadway Book with the child and parent together. The goal is the same as the last session's, except now the focus is on Sessions 7–11. Remember to cover each page carefully. Offer lots of praise for the child's accomplishments. This may be a more distressing activity than last session because you will be reviewing the more difficult graded exposure practice sessions and homework. This process should take 5–15 minutes.

Homework

Explain that the caregiver and the child need to pick another real-life exposure to practice for homework—ideally a more difficult item than last week. The child needs to stay with the situation until the anxiety goes down to a rating of 1. Practice the item once in the next week. Give them the filled out Parent Handout 11.1: Homework Check Sheet.

Preview the Next Session

Next week is the final session and the graduation ceremony.

Graduation

✓ *Review the Roadway Book.*
✓ *Lead graduation discussion.*

About This Session

You and the mother will likely feel a sense of accomplishment during this session. You will be able to compare, silently, how far the child has come since the first session. The graduation certificate will symbolize all of the hard work and the risks taken during therapy sessions and the *in vivo* exposures. The child will proudly (you hope) take home his or her decorated and personalized Roadway Book.

Materials

- Graduation diploma.
- Special snack.

Conducting the Session

Parent and Child Welcome

Child and parent are together for this session. Explain the plan for today. The main job is to review the Roadway Book, followed by a special snack and a little playtime, if desired.

Review the Last Session and the Homework

Review how the homework went. Did the child practice the real-life exposure? Take more than the usual 5 minutes if needed, because you will not split up and talk about it separately today.

The Roadway Book

The goal is to review every single page of Sessions 1–11. There are approximately 18 pages that span at least 3 months. As usual, the therapist is ultimately in charge of exploring the pages and turning to the next one at an appropriate pace. Try to have the child remember what the drawings on each page depict and what he or she learned. Try to go through the Roadway Book page by page and narrate the story from beginning to end. If the child is reluctant or tries to breeze over pages too fast, intervene by prompting, speaking for the child, or slowing him or her down, as appropriate.

If the child can't, or won't, recall, the therapist must verbalize it. Use lots of praise for the child's accomplishments. This should take 15 or more minutes.

There may or may not be compelling reasons to spend individual time with the mother. If needed, the end of this session can be used for that.

Graduation Diploma

Present a decorated graduation diploma. Break out the special snack.

Sign the diploma. From past mistakes, we've learned that the children really like the diploma *signed*; an unsigned diploma is rather disappointing.

Free electronic versions of a diploma can be found on the Internet fairly easily via search engines. Each clinic or practitioner will have to find his or her own version for personal use. Our diploma states:

Tulane University

This diploma is presented on
[Date], to

[Child's Name]

for successfully completing
the cognitive-behavioral therapy protocol
that includes recognizing feelings,
learning relaxation skills, and self-control of behavior.

_____

Therapist signature

Homework

None.

PART III

Parent Handouts, Child Worksheets, and Therapist Forms

Parent Handouts and Child Worksheets

Overview of the 12 Treatment Sessions

Session Number	Session Topics	Goals and Tasks
1	Education about PTSD Overview of the 12 sessions	Motivation/compliance
2	Oppositional defiant targets Parental leniency Make discipline plan	Plan for grief, if appropriate Address reluctance
3	Identify stressful feelings	Address reluctance
4	Learn scary feelings score Learn relaxation exercises	Address reluctance
5	Tell the story Create a stimulus hierarchy	Explore the caregiver's own trauma history and current symptoms Address reluctance
6	Easy narrative exposure Safety planning	Follow up with the caregiver Address reluctance
7	Medium narrative exposure Safety planning	Follow up with the caregiver Address reluctance
8	Medium narrative exposure Safety planning	Follow up with the caregiver Address reluctance
9	Worst-moment narrative exposure Safety planning	Follow up with the caregiver Address reluctance
10	Worst-moment narrative exposure Start review of the Roadway Book	Follow up with the caregiver Address reluctance
11	Learn relapse prevention	Review the Roadway Book
12	Review the Roadway Book	Graduation

Posttraumatic Stress Disorder (PTSD)

PTSD is a syndrome that some people get after they experience a life-threatening trauma.

WHAT IS A TRAUMA?

A trauma is something that is *life-threatening or threatens serious harm*. People can be traumatized by just witnessing something happen to someone else. Here is a list of types of traumas:

- Physical abuse
- Sexual abuse
- Serious accidents, such as car crashes
- Dog or large-animal attacks
- Seeing someone stabbed, shot, or killed
- Seeing one's mother beaten

WHAT ARE THE SYMPTOMS?

There are three categories of symptoms:

1. Reexperiencing Symptoms
   Children cannot stop thinking about the bad event, even if they want to. These symptoms may include:
   - Nightmares
   - Intrusive daydreams
   - Playing games that repeatedly reenact the trauma
   - Flashbacks
   - Getting very upset if something happens that reminds them of the trauma
   - Getting physically worked up by the reminders, including sweating, shaking, and fast heart rate

2. Numbing and Avoidance Symptoms
   Children emotionally shut down and try to avoid any reminders of what happened. These types of symptoms include:
   - Avoiding places or things that remind them of the trauma
   - Withdrawing from people
   - Looking less happy and acting less loving
   - Playing less than before

3. Increased Arousal Symptoms
   Children are more agitated and restless. These types of symptoms include:
   - Difficulty sleeping
   - Difficulty concentrating
   - Irritability, temper tantrums
   - More aggressive behaviors
   - More jumpy and scared

About You

My name is: _____

I am _____ years old

My family:

_____

_____

_____

My favorite game is: _____

My favorite TV show is: _____

My favorite color is: _____

The scary thing that happened to me was:

_____

_____

_____

_____

Changing My Thoughts

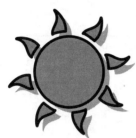 Parents' guilt may lead them to being too lenient, so that discipline is not enforced or consistent. Young children need consistent, loving discipline.

If you have been too lenient because you feel guilty about what has happened or feel sorry for your child, admitting this guilt is the first step. The second step is changing or replacing the thought that you are guilty. This technique is a well-known cognitive therapy strategy. This week we will work on changing your maladaptive thoughts for more appropriate thoughts. For example: Instead of thinking "Poor thing, he [she] has been through enough" (and then you don't discipline your child), think "Poor thing—but she [he] still has to follow the rules" (and then you follow through with appropriate discipline).

Step 1: What is your guilty thought?

_____

Step 2: What is a more appropriate thought that you can say to yourself?

 (Cut out the appropriate thought in the next box and place the paper in your wallet, on the fridge in the kitchen, or someplace where you will see it every day.)

I need to remember to say to myself:

_____

_____

Behaviors to Change

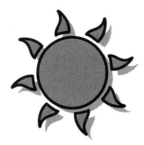

List of defiant behaviors to target for change:

1. _____

2. _____

3. _____

Discipline Plan for Defiant Behaviors

Target Behavior: _____

_____

_____

Sun.	Mon.	Tue.	Wed.	Thurs.	Fri.	Sat.
Sticker or ✓	Sticker or ✓	Sticker or ✓	Sticker or ✓	Sticker or ✓	Sticker or ✓	Sticker or ✓

Need to comply for _____ out of _____ days for . . .

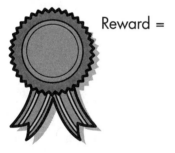 Reward =

Feelings in My Body

Draw the feelings in your body.

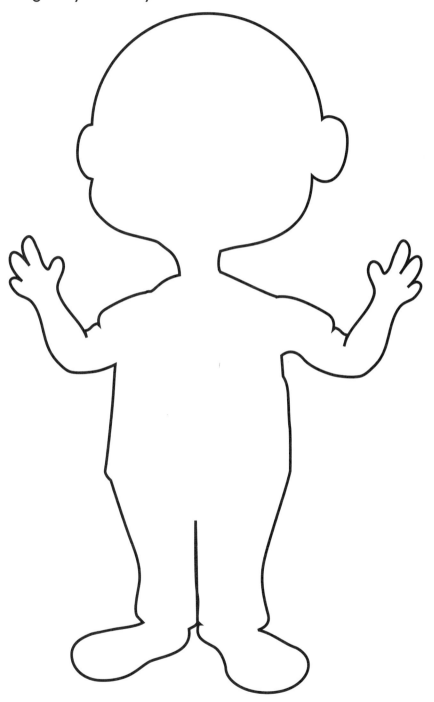

Homework: How Much I'm Scared

Plan: _____

Day/Time: _____

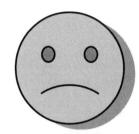

3. A lot

(Don't do this yet.)

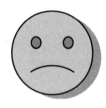

2. Medium

Aim for this one.

1. A little

0. None

Place Sticker Here:

Happy-Place Drawing

Draw your happy place.

Scary Feelings Score

Stressor: _____

3. A lot 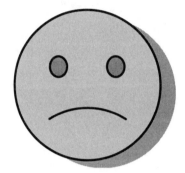 _____

2. Medium 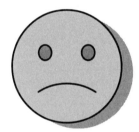 _____

1. A little   _____

0. None

Homework Check Sheet: Practice Once, Scary Feelings Score

Plan: _____

Day/Time: _____

3. A lot

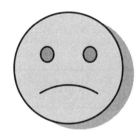

2. Medium

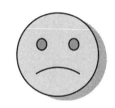   Aim for this one.

1. A little

0. None

Place Sticker Here:

The Whole Story about What Happened

DETAILS OF THE WHOLE STORY

What Happened:

_____

_____

_____

_____

_____

_____

_____

_____

When: _____

Who: _____

Where: _____

See: _____

Hear: _____

Smell: _____

Taste: _____

Touch: _____

Feelings: _____

Stimulus Hierarchy

FROM THE NOT TOO SCARY TO THE MOST SCARY

Most Scary:

Almost the Most Scary:

Medium Scary:

Medium Scary:

Not Too Scary:

Respecting Boundaries

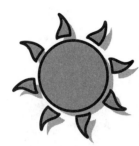

Sometimes parents' enthusiasm to help their children heal from trauma can unintentionally lead them to infringe on their children's privacy. Respecting your child's need for privacy will improve his/her response to therapy. This is often accomplished by ensuring a safe emotional space for the child to share feelings by not pushing the child to share what he/she is learning with others.

(Cut out the appropriate boundaries in the following box and place the paper in your wallet, on the fridge in the kitchen, or someplace where you will see it every day.)

What are some appropriate ways to support my child's healing while respecting his/her privacy boundaries?

_____

_____

Homework: Am I respecting my child's boundaries concerning his/her therapy and trauma recovery?

_____

_____

Homework Check Sheet: Practice Real-Life Exposure Once to Something Not Too Scary during the Next Week

Plan: _____

Day/Time: _____

How scared did you get?

3. A lot

2. Medium

1. A little

0. None

Write down what you really did:

Place Sticker Here:

Not-Too-Scary Reminder

Draw a not-too-scary reminder.

My Safety Plan

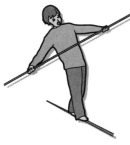

Danger Signs

1. _____

2. _____

3. _____

My Safety Plan:

Homework Check Sheet: Practice Real-Life Medium-Scary Exposure Once during the Next Week

Plan: _____

Day/Time: _____

How scared did you get?

3. A lot

2. Medium

1. A little

0. None

Write down what you really did:

Place Sticker Here:

Medium-Scary Reminder

Draw a medium-scary reminder.

Homework Check Sheet: Practice Real-Life Medium-Scary Exposure Once during the Next Week

Plan: _____

Day/Time: _____

How scared did you get?

3. A lot

2. Medium

1. A little

0. None

Write down what you really did:

Place Sticker Here:

Medium-Scary Reminder

Draw a medium-scary reminder.

My Safety Plan

Did you practice your Safety Plan?   Circle: Yes   or   No

If yes, congratulations!

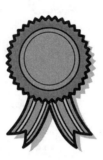

If no, practice now!

My Official Safety Plan:

_____

_____

_____

_____

_____

_____

_____

Homework Check Sheet: Practice Real-Life Almost-Too-Scary or Most-Scary Exposure Once during the Next Week

Plan: _____

Day/Time: _____

How scared did you get?

3. A lot

2. Medium

1. A little

0. None

Write down what you really did:

Place Sticker Here:

Worst-Moment Reminder

Draw a worst-moment reminder.

Homework Check Sheet: Practice Real-Life Almost-Too-Scary or Most-Scary Exposure Once during the Next Week

Plan: _____

Day/Time: _____

How scared did you get?

3. A lot

2. Medium

1. A little

0. None

Write down what you really did:

Place Sticker Here:

Worst-Moment Reminder

Draw a worst-moment reminder.

Homework Check Sheet: Practice Real-Life Almost-Too-Scary or Most-Scary Exposure Once during the Next Week

Plan: _____

Day/Time: _____

How scared did you get?

3. A lot

2. Medium

1. A little

0. None

Write down what you really did:

Place Sticker Here:

Near-Future Reminder

Draw a child in the near future and a reminder.

Distant-Future Reminder

Draw a child as an adult and a reminder.

Reluctance Checklist

Today's Date: _____   Session No.: _____

How Reluctant Did the *Parent* Feel before Coming to Today's Session?

"How strongly did you consider not coming today?"

0	1	2	3	4	5	6	7	8	9	10

None   A little   Medium   Extreme

Comparison to   Clean the   Go to the   Public
other things: dishes   dentist   speaking

Why Did the *Parent* Not Want to Come to Today's Session?

None   A little   A lot

0	1	2	Thought child would be distressed.
0	1	2	Thought parent would be distressed.
0	1	2	Believed child improved enough/didn't need more therapy.
0	1	2	Believed child was not improving/this was a waste of time.
0	1	2	Not enough time for this because of other life pressures.
0	1	2	Other: _____

How Reluctant Did the *Child* Feel before Coming to Today's Session?

"How strongly did your child consider not coming today?"

0	1	2	3	4	5	6	7	8	9	10

None   A little   Medium   Extreme

Comparison to   Brush teeth   Go to the   Homework   Eat vegetables
other things: dentist

Why Did the *Child* Not Want to Come to Today's Session?

None   A little   A lot

0	1	2	Thought he/she would be distressed.
0	1	2	Thought parent would be distressed.
0	1	2	Believed he/she had improved enough/didn't need more therapy.
0	1	2	Believed he/she was not improving/this was a waste of time.
0	1	2	Not enough time for this because of other interests.
0	1	2	Other: _____

The Relaxing Two-Step Exercises

These simple relaxation exercises are for young children. All of the steps are in two's so that children can remember how to complete each exercise. When teaching these exercises, the instructor should do each one with the child so that he or she understands the steps. Have the child practice each exercise with the caregiver and on his or her own.

Encourage the child to go through the imagery, breathing, and muscle relaxation exercises. If the child prefers one exercise more than the others, that's OK too.

After children have mastered each exercise, they may want to make up their own "Fun, Two-Step Exercise," using their own fun moves as a way to be silly and interact with the teaching adult.

Imagery

1. Close your eyes.

2. Imagine yourself in a happy, safe place or at a happy, safe event (15–30 seconds).

Breathing—Repeat Twice

1. Breathe in slowly through your nose and fill your belly with air, like a balloon (in for two counts, hold for two, blow out for two).

2. Breathe in slowly again through your nose and fill your belly with air, like a balloon (in for two counts, hold for two, blow out for two).

Muscle Relaxation—Repeat Twice

1. Tighten your arm muscles (hold for two counts) and then let your arms fall loose like noodles.

2. Tighten your arm muscles again (hold for two counts) and then let your arms fall like looseynoodles.

***Optional Stretching**—Repeat Twice*

Stretch up ("Reach for the stars") and relax.

Written for PPT by Alison Salloum.

Scary Feelings Score Form

Write the child's scary feelings score (1, 2, or 3) in the boxes below. Check every 3–5 minutes. The exposure does not have to last 10 minutes, or it can last longer. Use the bottom or the back of this sheet if more columns are needed.

	Minutes since Exposure Started										
	Base-line 0	1	2	3	4	5	6	7	8	9	10
Session 5: Telling the Story											
Session 6: Easy Exposure											
Session 7: Medium Exposure											
Session 8: Medium Exposure											
Session 9: Worst Exposure											
Session 10: Worst Exposure											

Illustrations of PTSD Symptoms

This set of 19 cartoons was modified from the Darryl cartoons created by Richard Neugebauer, PhD. The original Darryl cartoons* depicted acts of community violence with one man assaulting another. I expanded this concept with the artist Carol Peebles, who modified the central boy character, added a central girl character, and drew the scenes of domestic violence and motor vehicle accidents. Other cartoons have since been created by others, as needed, by tracing or mimicking her work as templates.

We used the cartoons with preschool-age children to educate them about PTSD symptoms, beginning with a clinical trial in 2005 (R34 MH70827) funded by the National Institute of Mental Health. Our main goal was to teach them that these behaviors are symptoms. This aim contrasts with the original purpose of the Neugebauer cartoons, which was to interview school-age children to find out if they had symptoms of PTSD (Neugebauer et al., 1999).

For the education process to work optimally, the cartoon trauma scenes need to be individualized to each child's personal trauma. That is why the Darryl scenes of community violence were not the best suited for children who had other types of traumatic experiences. If a child with whom you are working has a trauma experience that does not match one of the scenes in these cartoons, you have my permission to replace the scenes in the thought bubbles with a drawing of your own. If you share your creation with anyone else, you must add in writing somehow on the cartoon that it was your modification so that none of us—Scheeringa, Peebles, or Neugebauer—is credited and/or held responsible for your effort.

---

* Available from Dr. Neugebauer, *rn3@columbia.edu*.

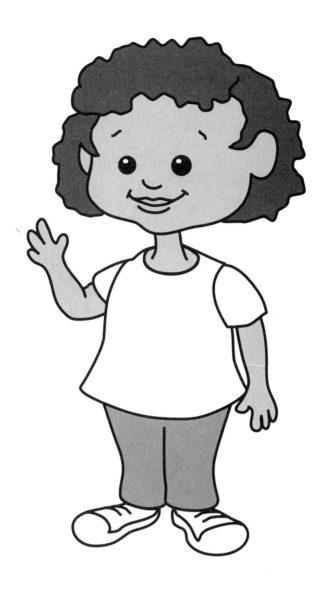

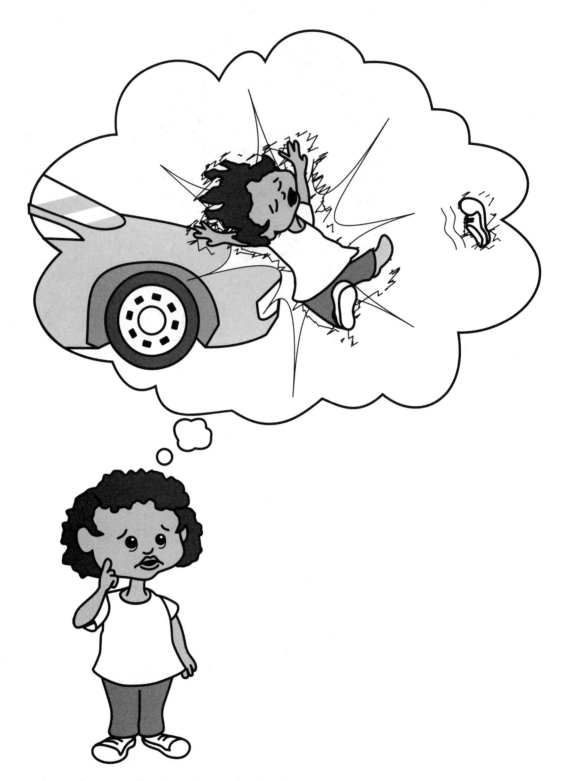

Intrusive recollections (i.e., thinks about it when she doesn't want to)

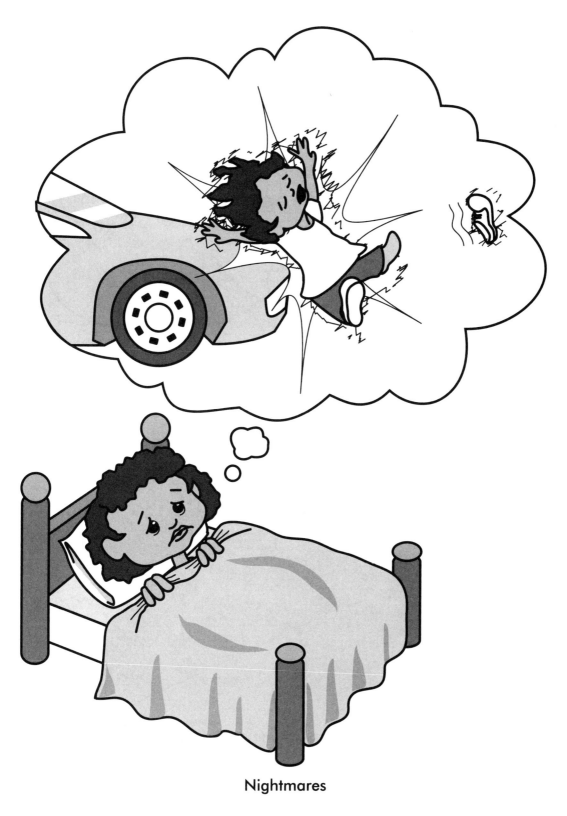

Nightmares

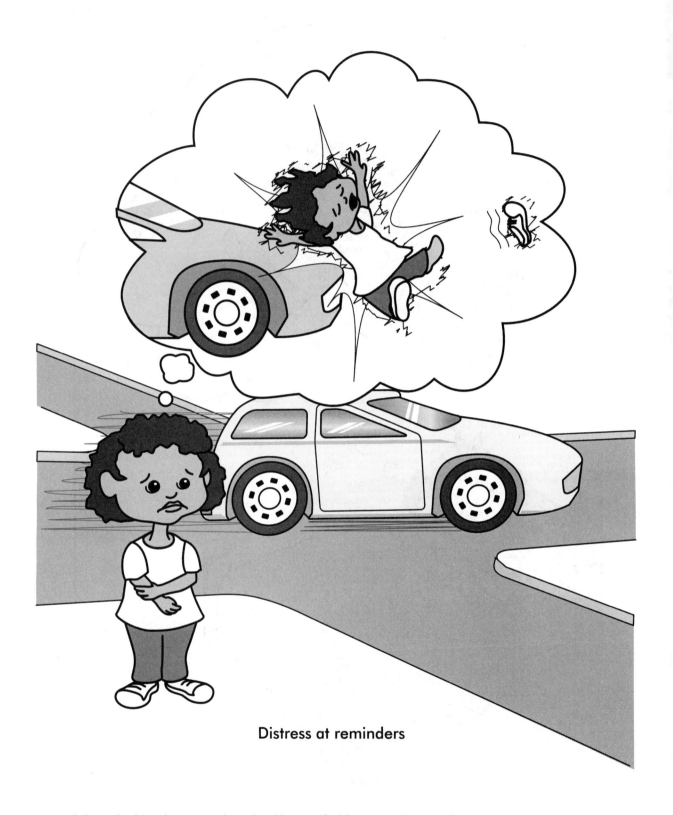

Distress at reminders

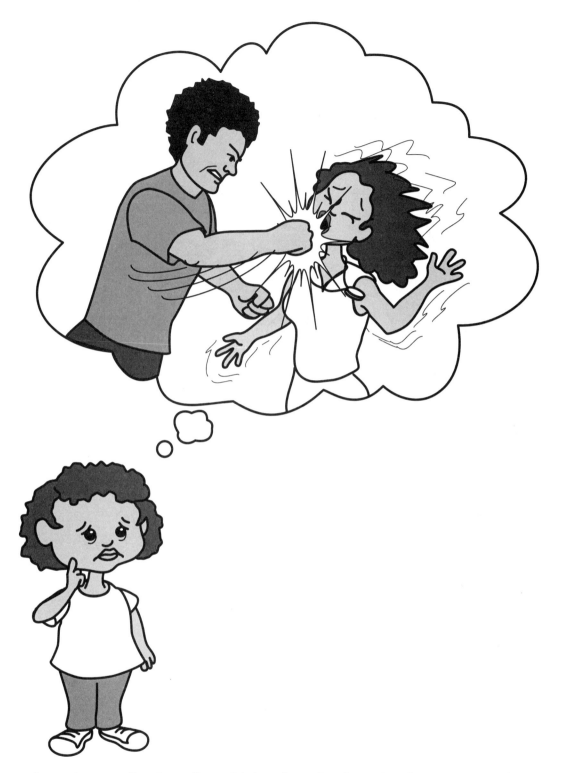

Intrusive recollections (i.e., thinks about it when she doesn't want to)

Copyright by Michael S. Scheeringa and Carol Peebles. Modified from Neugebauer et al. (1999).

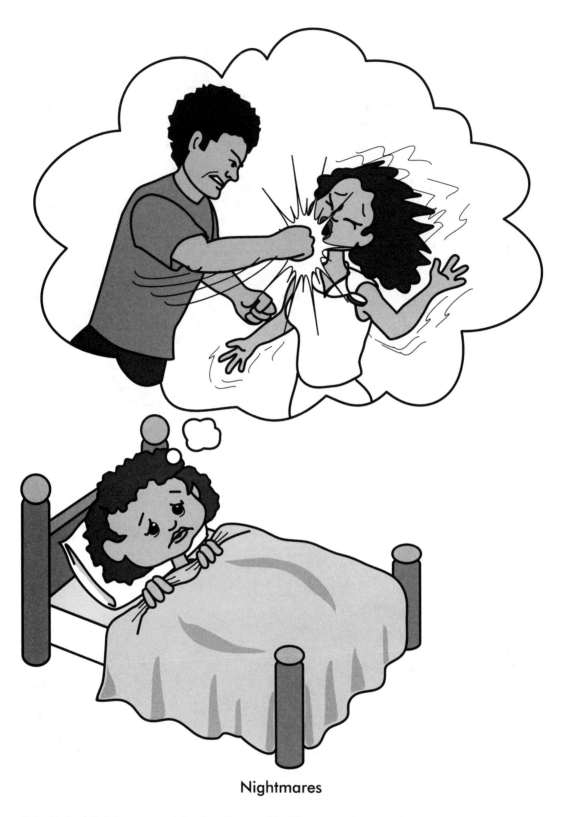

Nightmares

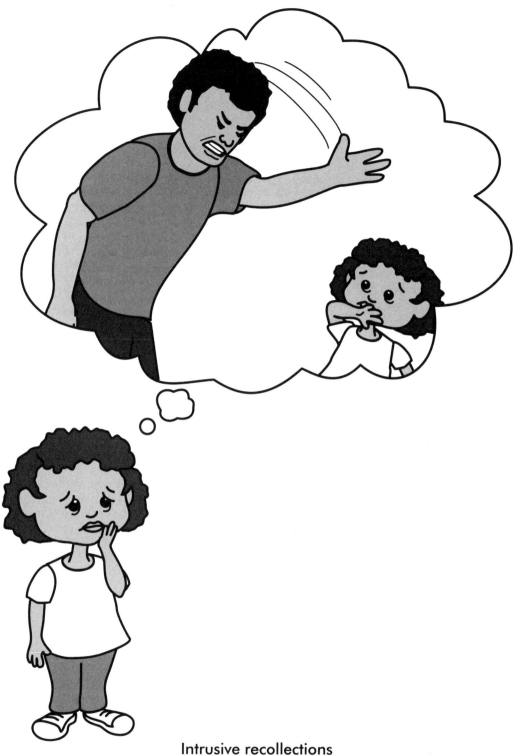

**Intrusive recollections
(i.e., thinks about it when she doesn't want to)**

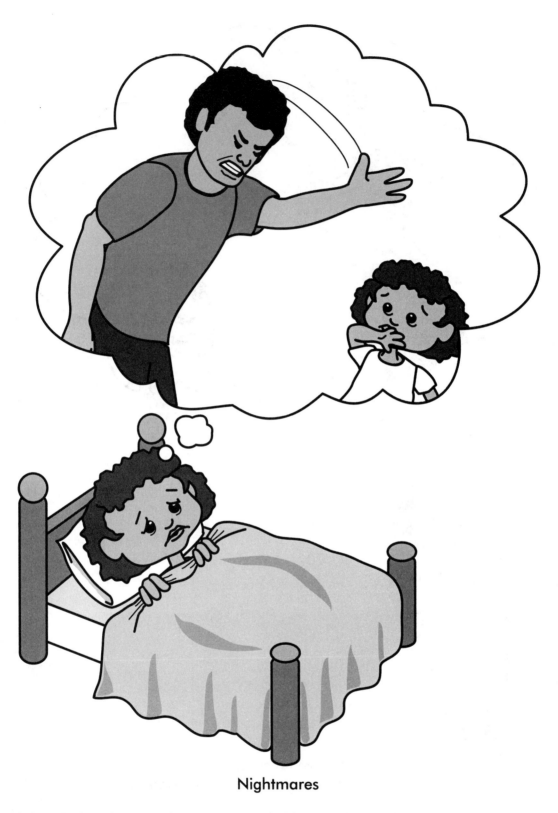

Nightmares

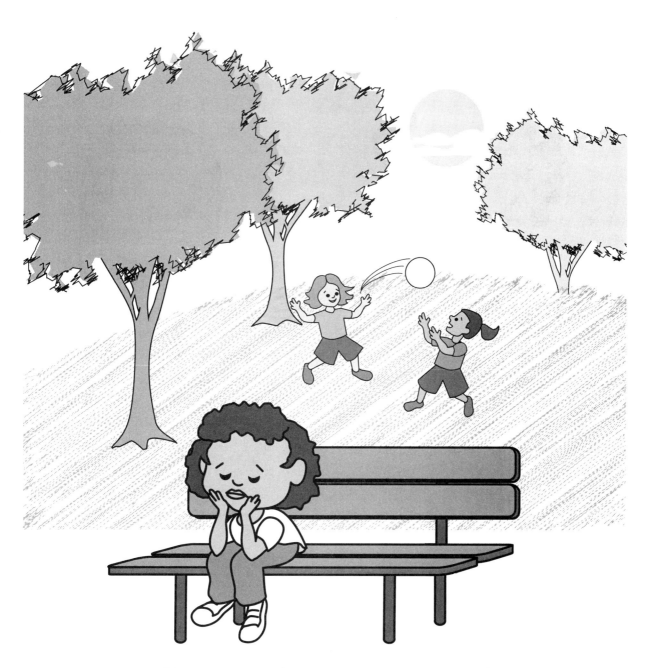

Loss of interest in usual activities (i.e., constriction of play)

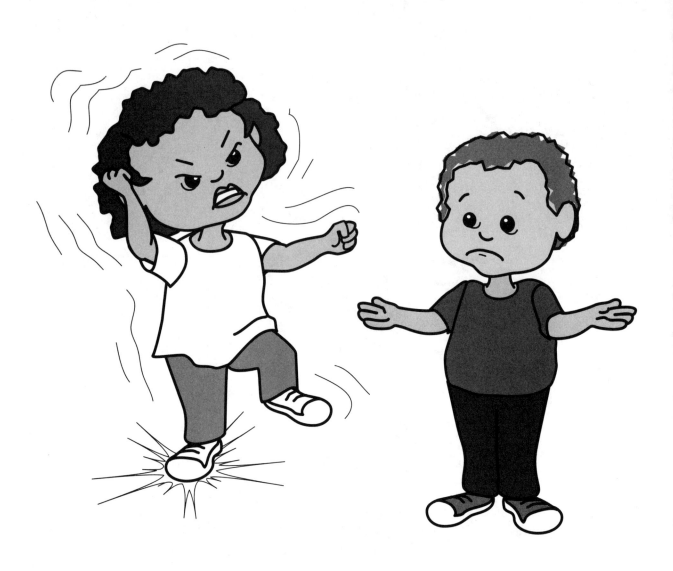

Irritability or outbursts of anger. Extreme temper tantrums.

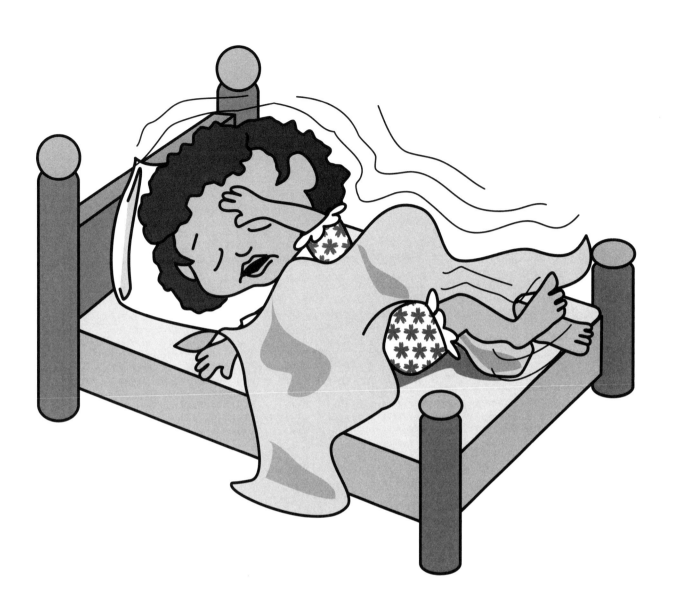

Difficulty sleeping

Copyright by Michael S. Scheeringa and Carol Peebles. Modified from Neugebauer et al. (1999).

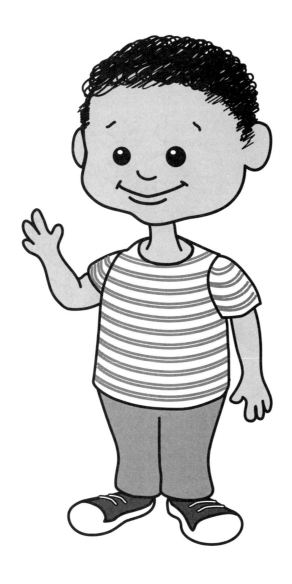

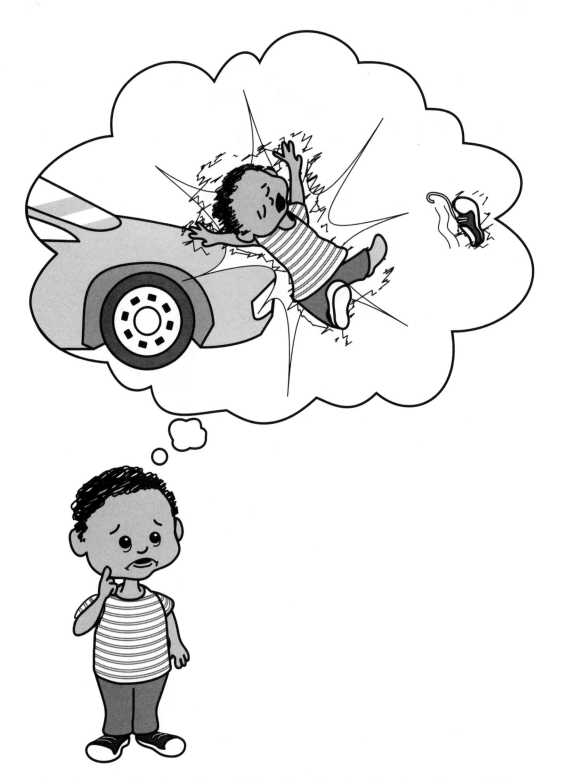

Intrusive recollections (i.e., thinks about it when he doesn't want to)

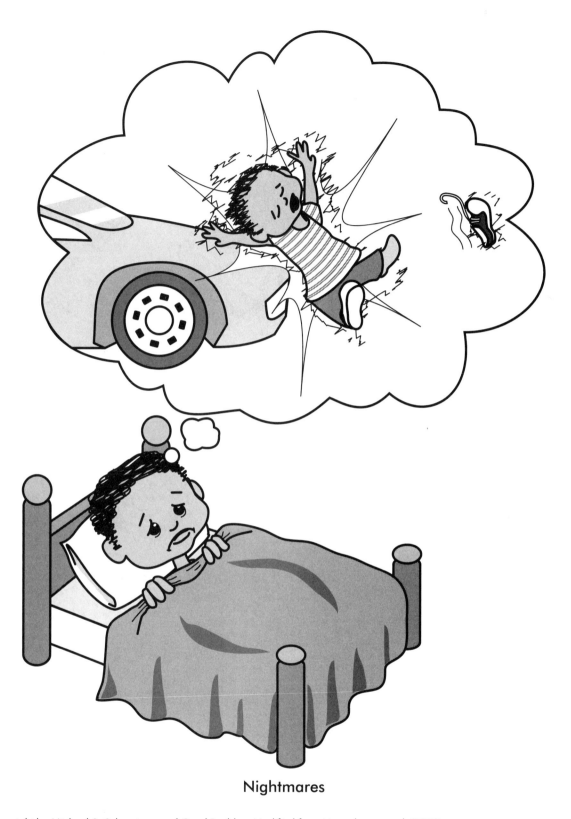

Nightmares

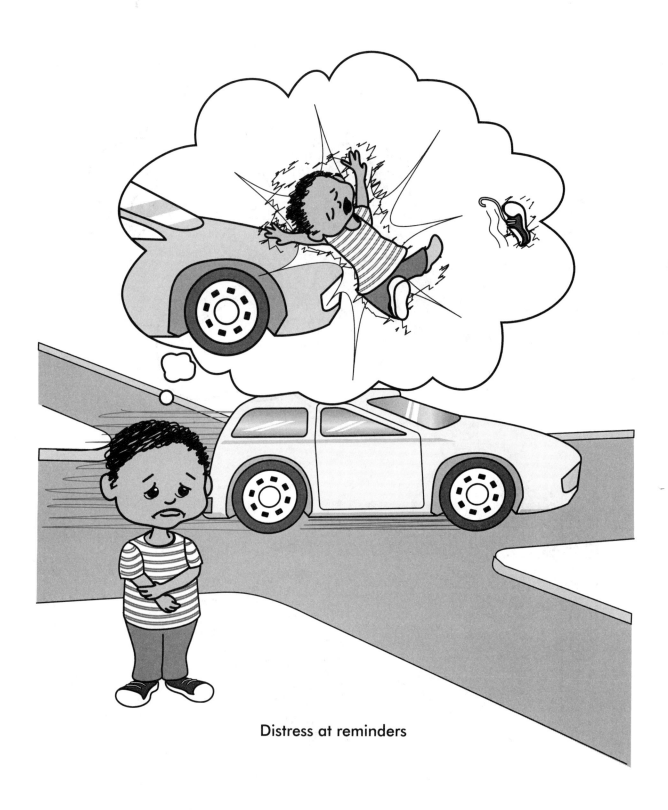

Distress at reminders

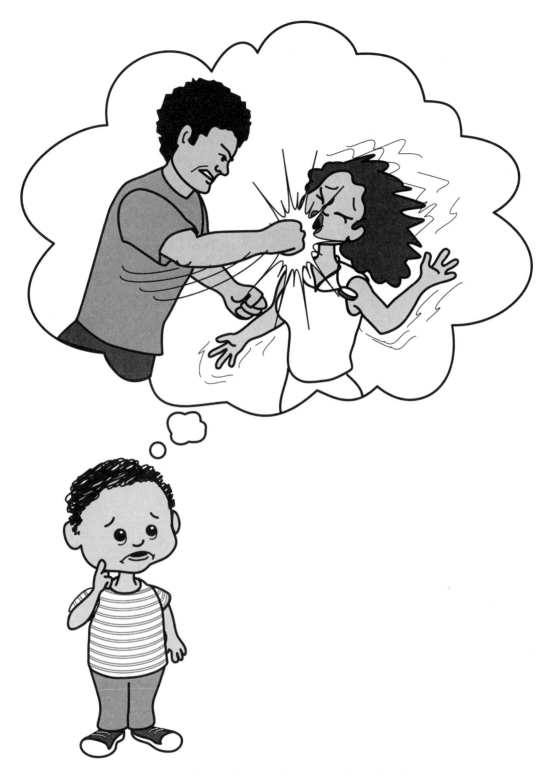

Intrusive recollections (i.e., thinks about it when he doesn't want to)

Copyright by Michael S. Scheeringa and Carol Peebles. Modified from Neugebauer et al. (1999).

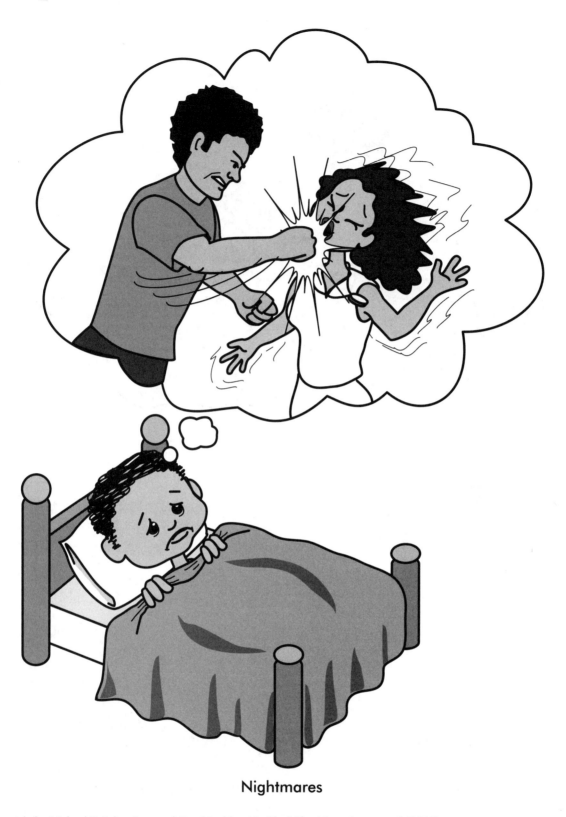

Nightmares

Copyright by Michael S. Scheeringa and Carol Peebles. Modified from Neugebauer et al. (1999).

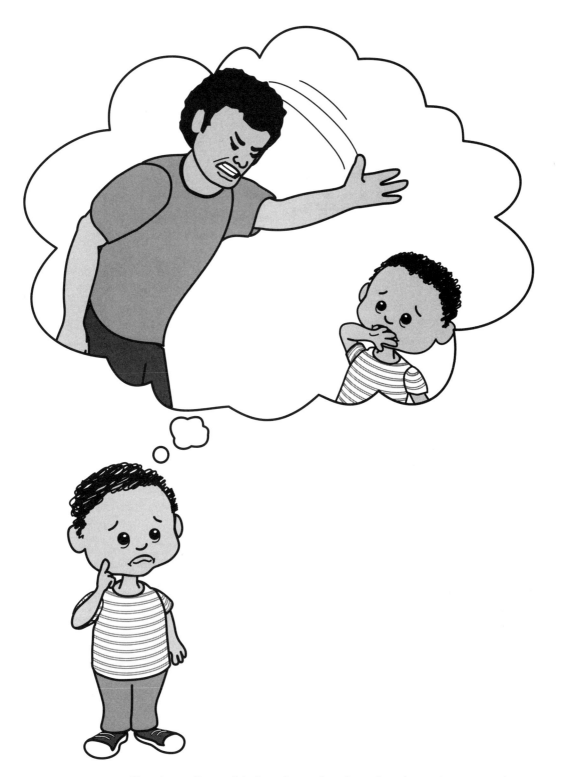

Intrusive recollections (i.e., thinks about it when he doesn't want to)

Copyright by Michael S. Scheeringa and Carol Peebles. Modified from Neugebauer et al. (1999).

From Michael S. Scheeringa (2016). Copyright by The Guilford Press. Permission to photocopy this material is granted to purchasers of this book for personal use only (see copyright page for details). Purchasers can download and print additional copies of this material (see the box at the end of the table of contents).

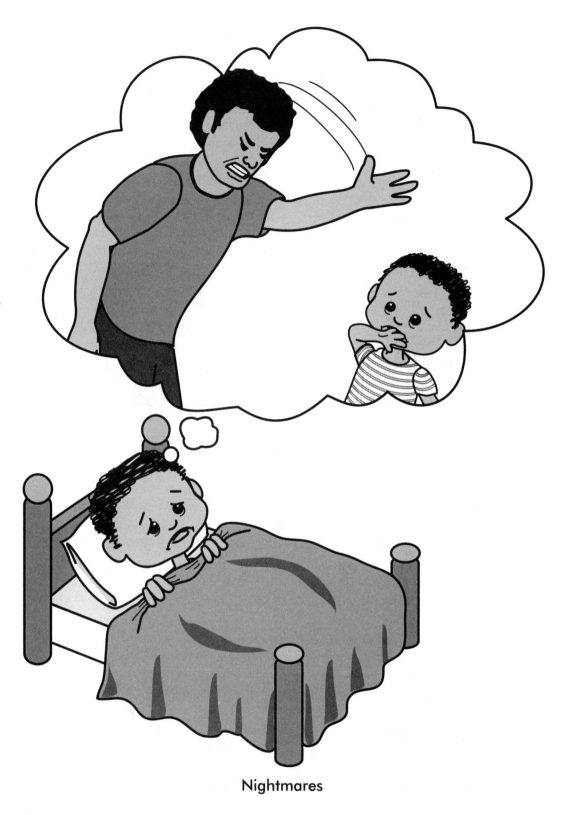

Nightmares

Copyright by Michael S. Scheeringa and Carol Peebles. Modified from Neugebauer et al. (1999).

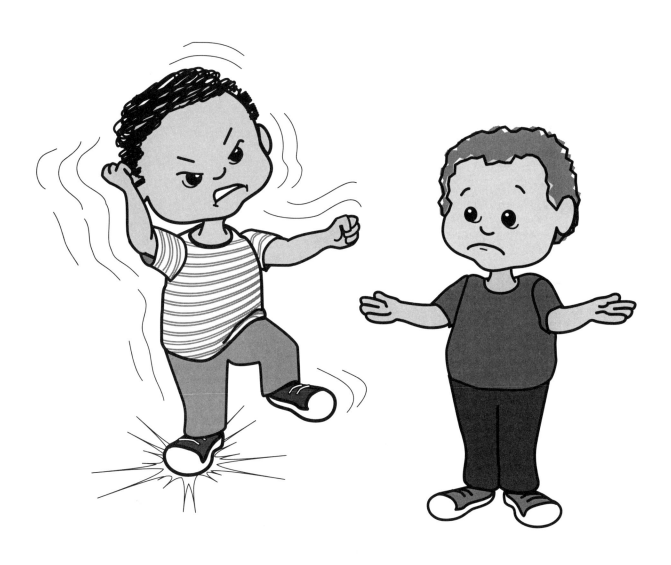

Irritability or outbursts of anger. Extreme temper tantrums.

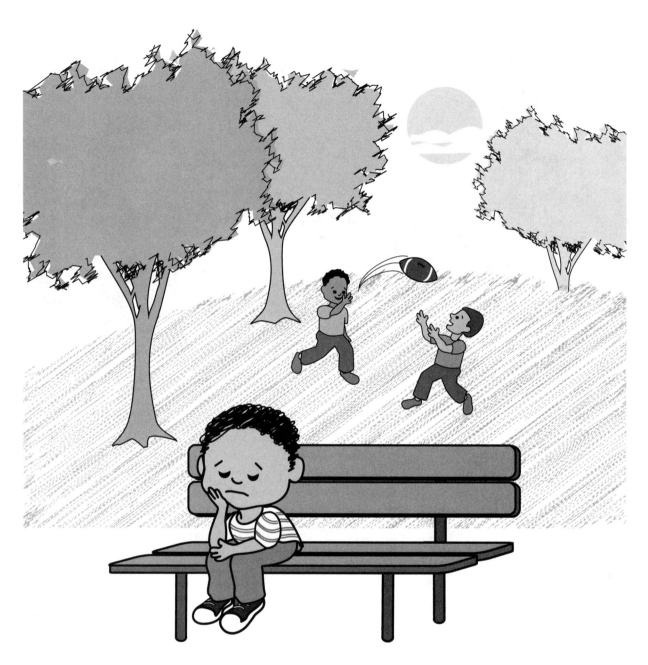

Loss of interest in usual activities (i.e., constriction of play)

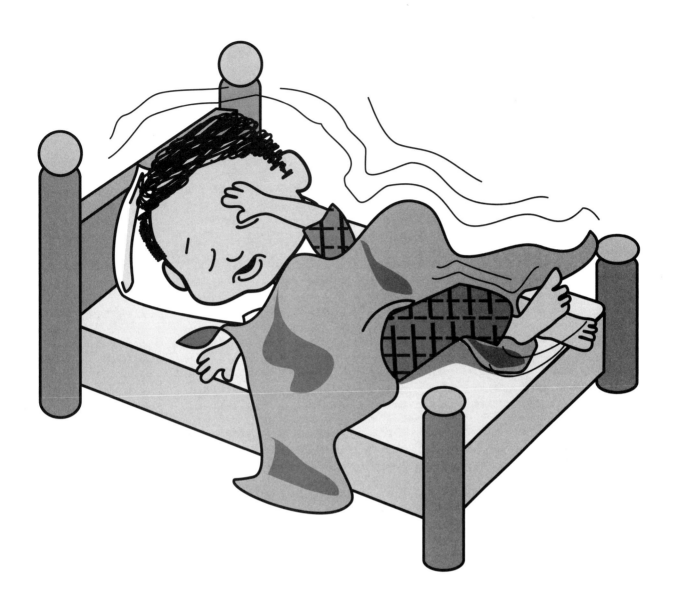

Difficulty sleeping

APPENDIX 2

Fidelity and Achievement ChecklisT (FACT)

For each of the 12 sessions, sets of tasks are listed to help therapists check (1) their fidelity to the manual and (2) how well children were able to complete the activities. This is the first fidelity checklist, to my knowledge, that measures how well children are able to complete the tasks. Therapists may attempt tasks with fidelity, but that does not measure whether children are able to do the tasks. When measuring fidelity to an evidence-based treatment, what children are able to do seems equally important as what therapists do.

Code these events for whenever they happen in the course of therapy, within your discretion of whether it makes sense. For example, if Session 3 had to be cut short due to time, and the therapist picked up in Session 4 with the end of Session 3 material, then it would make sense to give the therapist credit for covering the material. Likewise, items can be endorsed if the therapist forgot to do something and then remembered to do it later, as long as it makes sense within the rest of the protocol.

0   Therapist or child did not attempt it.

1   Therapist or child attempted it partially.

2   Therapist or child fully completed the therapeutic technique. Partial or questionable attempts do not count.

When rating therapists, if the children or caregivers did not seem to comprehend the construct, this does not count against the therapist. Code for the therapist's attempts, not the effectiveness.

THERAPIST

____ Explained the concept of PTSD to the caregiver and child together.

____ Defined life-threatening traumas to the caregiver and child together.

____ Defined the three types of symptoms—reexperiencing, avoidance/numbing, and increased arousal—to the caregiver and child together.

____ Gave handout on PTSD to the caregiver to take home.

____ Used cartoons to explain several PTSD symptoms to the child.

____ Explained the routine of splitting up for future sessions.

____ Introduced the Roadway Book and allowed the child to personalize it.

____ Had the child attempt the first Roadway Book assignment.

____ Introduced the topic of resistance/reluctance to the caregiver.

____ Explained that reluctance can be normal.

____ Assured the caregiver that reluctance typically decreases with therapy and time.

CHILD

____ From verbal discussion and the handout (not with the cartoons), the child appeared to understand the concept of PTSD as something that has impacted on him or her.

____ The child appeared to understand the PTSD symptoms that were presented with the cartoons.

____ The child completed first worksheet for the Roadway Book.

SESSION 2

THERAPIST

____ Reviewed the last session with the caregiver and child together.

____ Defined oppositional and defiant behavior.

____ Discussed the theory that caregivers may feel guilty and become lenient with discipline.

____ Negotiated an agreement with the caregiver about the cause of child's defiant behavior.

____ Made a priority list of defiant behaviors that the caregiver wants to reduce.

____ Created a discipline plan with a daily reward.

____ Asked the caregiver to rate her reluctance prior to coming to the appointment on a scale of 1–10.

____ Asked the caregiver what "tricks" she used to overcome her reluctance. If there was no reluctance, code *1* here.

____ Reminded the caregiver that the reluctance may get worse. If there was no reluctance, the therapist must still do this to score *1*.

____ Sent child and caregiver home with a homework sheet.

CHILD

____ Understood that he or she has been oppositional in relation to Mother's house rules. (The child does not need to agree to change the behavior.)

____ Understood the new homework assignment on the behavioral plan.

SESSION 3

THERAPIST

____ Reviewed the last session with the child.

____ Encouraged the child to draw feelings on body outline drawing.

____ Attempted the worksheet for Session 3 in the Roadway Book.

____ Reviewed the last session with the caregiver.

____ Inquired whether the feelings that the child revealed were new to the caregiver.

____ Asked the caregiver to rate her reluctance prior to coming to appointment on a scale of 1–10.

____ Asked the caregiver what "tricks" she used to overcome her reluctance. If there was no reluctance, code 1 here.

____ Explained the homework to the caregiver and child.

____ Reminded the caregiver that the reluctance may get worse.

____ Sent child and caregiver home with homework sheet.

CHILD

____ Completed body drawing with feelings.

____ Able to talk about feelings without reference to the body drawing.

____ Practiced relaxation techniques.

____ Understood new homework assignment on practicing relaxation technique daily.

SESSION 4

THERAPIST

____ Reviewed homework with the caregiver and child.

____ Reviewed the last session with the child.

____ Taught relaxation techniques with all three parts: (1) imaginary happy place, (2) slowed and paced breathing, and (3) muscle relaxation.

____ Explained the scary feelings score, including the worksheet.

____ Reviewed the last session with the caregiver.

____ Reviewed the relaxation techniques with the caregiver.

____ Explained the scary feelings score to the caregiver, including the worksheet.

____ Asked the caregiver to rate her reluctance prior to coming to appointment on a scale of 1–10.

____ Asked the caregiver what "tricks" she used to overcome her reluctance. If there was no reluctance, code 1 here.

____ Reminded the caregiver that the reluctance may get worse. If there was no reluctance, the therapist must at least verbally note this to score 1.

____ Explained the homework and gave the caregiver the homework check sheet.

CHILD

____ Completed the homework for last week.

____ Remembered what his or her homework assignment had been (prompts from the therapist are allowable).

____ Completed the scary feelings score worksheet.

____ Understood the new homework assignment of identifying a stressful time next week, rating it on the scary feelings score, and practicing relaxation.

THERAPIST

____ Discussed the old homework with the caregiver and child at the beginning.

____ Encouraged the child to tell the whole trauma story from start to finish.

____ Asked the child to rate his or her anxiety on the scary feelings score more than once.

____ Had the child attempt one or more relaxation exercises at least once.

____ Attempted to create a stimulus hierarchy list.

____ Allowed the caregiver an open-ended opportunity to talk about what she had just heard from her child or to talk about her own feelings and memories.

____ Asked the caregiver if her distress is perceptible to her child.

____ Asked the caregiver to rate her reluctance prior to coming to appointment on a scale of 1–10.

____ Asked the caregiver what "tricks" she used to overcome her reluctance. If there was no reluctance, code *1* here.

____ Reminded the caregiver that the reluctance may get worse. If there was no reluctance, the therapist must at least verbally note this to score *1*.

____ Explained the homework to the caregiver and gave her the homework check sheet.

CHILD

____ Remembered what his or her homework assignment had been (prompts from the therapist are allowable).

____ Completed the homework for last week.

____ Recounted his or her trauma story with at least three details.

____ Identified at least three aspects of the trauma as distinct upsetting events (for the stimulus hierarchy list).

____ Understood the new homework assignment of practicing imaginal exposure and relaxation once next week.

THERAPIST

____ Discussed the old homework with the caregiver and child at the beginning.

____ Started drawing/imaginal exposure with an easy item from the stimulus hierarchy list, including drawing for the Roadway Book.

____ Asked the child to his or her rate anxiety with a scary feelings score more than once during the exposure.

____ Had the child attempt one or more relaxation exercise at least once.

____ Introduced safety planning to the child, including the concepts of danger signals and making a plan.

____ Addressed safety planning with the child.

____ Asked the caregiver her thoughts after watching the child's sessions.

____ Reviewed the safety plan concepts with the caregiver.

____ Asked the caregiver to rate her reluctance prior to coming to appointment on a scale of 1–10.

____ Asked the caregiver what "tricks" she used to overcome her reluctance. If there was no reluctance, code 1 here.

____ Reminded the caregiver that the reluctance may get worse. If there was no reluctance, the therapist must at least verbally note this to score 1.

____ Explained the homework to the caregiver and gave her the homework check sheet.

CHILD

____ Completed the homework for last week.

____ Completed the drawing exposure of an easy task from the stimulus hierarchy list.

____ Completed the imaginal exposure of an easy task from the stimulus hierarchy list.

____ Brought his or her anxiety down to at least a rating of 2 on the scary feelings score before the end of the session.

____ Understood the new homework assignment of an easy *in vivo* exposure practice.

____ Understood the safety plan.

SESSION 7

THERAPIST

____ Reviewed the old homework with the caregiver and child.

____ Attempted drawing/imaginal exposure with a medium item from the stimulus hierarchy list, including drawing for the Roadway Book.

____ Asked the child to rate his or her anxiety with a scary feelings score more than once during exposure.

____ Had the child attempt one or more relaxation exercises at least once.

____ Addressed safety planning with the child.

____ Asked the caregiver for her thoughts after watching the child's sessions.

____ Addressed safety planning with the caregiver.

____ Asked the caregiver to rate her reluctance prior to coming to the appointment on a scale of 1–10.

____ Asked the caregiver what "tricks" she used to overcome her reluctance. If there was no reluctance, code 1 here.

____ Reminded the caregiver that the reluctance may get worse. If there was no reluctance, the therapist must at least verbally note this to score 1.

____ Explained the homework to the caregiver and child together and gave the caregiver the homework check sheet.

CHILD

____ Completed the homework for last week.

____ Completed the drawing exposure of a medium task from the stimulus hierarchy list.

____ Completed the imaginal exposure of a medium task from the stimulus hierarchy list.

____ Brought his or her anxiety down to at least a rating of 2 on the scary feelings score before the end of the session.

____ Understood the new homework assignment of a medium *in vivo* exposure practice.

____ Understood the safety plan.

SESSION 8

THERAPIST

____ Reviewed the old homework with the caregiver and child.

____ Attempted the drawing/imaginal exposure with a medium item from the stimulus hierarchy list, including drawing for the Roadway Book.

____ Asked child to rate his or her anxiety with a scary feelings score more than once during the exposure.

____ Had the child attempt one or more relaxation exercises at least once.

____ Addressed safety planning with the child.

____ Asked the caregiver for her thoughts after watching the child's sessions.

____ Addressed safety planning with the caregiver.

____ Asked the caregiver to rate her reluctance prior to coming to appointment on a scale of 1–10.

____ Asked the caregiver what "tricks" she used to overcome her reluctance. If there was no reluctance, code *1* here.

____ Reminded the caregiver that the reluctance may get worse. If there was no reluctance, the therapist must at least verbally note this to score *1*.

____ Explained the homework to the caregiver and the child and gave the caregiver the homework check sheet.

CHILD

____ Completed the homework for last week.

____ Completed the drawing exposure of a medium task from the stimulus hierarchy list.

____ Completed the imaginal exposure of a medium task from the stimulus hierarchy list.

____ Brought his or her anxiety down to at least a rating of 2 on the scary feelings score before the end of the session.

____ Understood the new homework assignment of a medium *in vivo* exposure practice.

____ Understood the safety plan.

THERAPIST

____ Reviewed the old homework with the caregiver and child.

____ Attempted the drawing/imaginal exposure with a worst-moment item from the stimulus hierarchy list, including drawing for the Roadway Book.

____ Asked the child to rate his or her anxiety with a scary feelings score more than once during the exposure.

____ Had the child attempt one or more relaxation exercises at least once.

____ Addressed safety planning with child.

____ Asked the caregiver for her thoughts after watching the child's sessions.

____ Addressed safety planning with the caregiver.

____ Asked the caregiver to rate her reluctance prior to coming to appointment on a scale of 1–10.

____ Asked the caregiver what "tricks" she used to overcome her reluctance. If there was no reluctance, code 1 here.

____ Explained the homework to the caregiver and child and gave the caregiver the homework check sheet.

CHILD

____ Completed the homework for last week.

____ Completed the drawing exposure of the worst moment from the stimulus hierarchy list.

____ Completed the imaginal exposure of the worst moment from the stimulus hierarchy list.

____ Brought his or her anxiety down to at least a rating of 2 on the scary feelings score before the end of the session.

____ Understood the new homework assignment of a hard *in vivo* exposure practice.

____ Understood the safety plan.

SESSION 10

THERAPIST

____ Reviewed the old homework with the caregiver and child.

____ Attempted the drawing/imaginal exposure with a worst-moment item from the stimulus hierarchy list, including drawing for the Roadway Book.

____ Asked the child to rate his or her anxiety with a scary feelings score more than once during exposure.

____ Had the child attempt one or more relaxation exercises at least once.

____ Asked the caregiver her thoughts after watching her child's sessions.

____ Started review of the Roadway Book with the dyad.

____ Asked the caregiver to rate her reluctance prior to coming to appointment on a scale of 1–10.

____ Asked the caregiver what "tricks" she used to overcome her reluctance. If there was no reluctance, code 1 here.

____ Explained the homework to the caregiver and child and gave the caregiver the homework check sheet.

____ Previewed with both that only two more sessions are left.

CHILD

____ Completed the homework for last week.

____ Remembered what his or her homework assignment had been (prompts from the therapist are allowable).

____ Completed the drawing exposure of the worst moment from the stimulus hierarchy list.

____ Completed the imaginal exposure of the worst moment from the stimulus hierarchy list.

____ Brought his or her anxiety down to at least a rating of 2 on the scary feelings score before the end of the session.

____ Understood the new homework assignment of a hard *in vivo* exposure practice.

THERAPIST

____ Reviewed the old homework with the caregiver and child.

____ Asked the child to think of events in the near future that might make bad memories pop back up. Asked the child to draw it.

____ Asked the child what tools he or she would use to handle those bad memories.

____ Asked the child to think of the future when grown up and a bad memory would pop up.

____ Asked the child what tools he or she would use to handle those bad memories.

____ Asked the child for current scary feelings score more than once.

____ Had the child attempt one or more relaxation exercises at least once.

____ Continued review of the Roadway Book with the dyad.

____ Reminded the caregiver that the next session is the last one.

____ Asked the caregiver to rate her reluctance prior to coming to appointment on a scale of 1–10.

____ Explained the homework to both and gave the caregiver the homework check sheet.

CHILD

____ Completed the homework for last week.

____ Remembered what his or her homework assignment had been (prompts from the therapist are allowable).

____ Able to talk about an event that could happen tomorrow and would bring back bad memories.

____ Completed the drawing worksheet on this topic.

____ Able to talk about an event that could happen in the distant future and would bring back bad memories.

____ Completed the drawing worksheet on this topic.

____ Brought his or her anxiety down to at least a rating of 2 on the scary feelings score before the end of their session.

____ Understood the new homework assignment of a hard *in vivo* exposure practice.

THERAPIST

____ Reviewed the old homework with the caregiver and child.

____ Attempted to review every page of the Roadway Book with the child and caregiver.

____ Presented graduation diploma.

CHILD

____ Completed the homework for last week.

____ Remembered what his or her homework assignment had been (prompts from the therapist are allowable).

____ Reviewed the Roadway Book.

Cheat Sheets

PARENT AND CHILD

1. Engage/introductions.

2. Offer candy—will be put away, but offered at the beginning of every session.

3. Describe purpose:
   - Deal with trauma and the symptoms of PTSD to feel better.
   - Make sure that the parent has told the child why they are coming to treatment.
   - Not getting shots or because they are bad.

4. Inform them of 12-session format:
   - Explain routine of splitting up the focus of sessions between child and mother.
   - Give mother outline of 12 sessions.

5. Explain the concept of PTSD scary thoughts/feelings to mother and child together:
   - Describe how we know traumas can cause symptoms in people.
   - Define a life-threatening trauma (use examples for adults and for kids).

6. Provide education on three types of symptoms to the child and mother together:
   - Reexperiencing, avoidance/numbing, and increased arousal.
   - Give handout for parents to read later about PTSD.
   - Use cartoons to create a brief story.
   - Check that child understands trauma impact on them, that this is bad, and that they want it to go away.
   - Point out that we will make the scary feelings/thoughts go away feel better.

7. Introduce the Roadway Book. Show the child the three-prong binder—explain it will be theirs to work on—like telling a story (beginning, middle, end); like a toolbox:
   - Allow child to personalize it. Write child's name on front cover and let child decorate it with stickers and markers.
   - Have child name the book; if cannot think of a name, call it the Roadway Book.

8. Complete the first assignment:
   - Allow child to draw and color on the worksheet. Ask questions to get answers for the worksheet items.
   - Tell child that their trauma is the scary event instead of asking them (can confirm unexpected answers later with parent).
   - Have extra paper ready for Tom Sawyer trick, if needed.

9. Preview next session with parent and child, including talking about behavior and creating a behavior plan.

10. Cover reluctance with parent:
    - Introduce topic of resistance/reluctance.
    - Explain that reluctance is normal and may increase over the course of therapy (if not, this is OK too); encourage the mother to continue to come even with reluctance.
    - Assure mother that reluctance typically decreases with therapy and time; you will check in about this at every session.

PARENT AND CHILD

1. Welcome; offer candy to child.

2. Review what has been learned so far: PTSD/scary feelings and the Roadway Book.

3. Explain defiance; briefly review data from the intake what the parent thought were problems.

4. Time course of defiance? Completely new or worse after the trauma?

5. Explain theory about guilt and leniency with discipline; ask parent if this accurate. If not, explore her reasoning; if so, move on to intervention.
   - Key is to negotiate an agreement with mother that she will work toward ignoring her guilt and empathy for the child and reinforce discipline.
   - Explain that this is a well-known cognitive therapy technique to recognize maladaptive thoughts and replace them with more appropriate thoughts.
   - Give an example: "Poor thing, he has been through so much." Replace with "Poor thing, he has been through so much, but he still has to follow the rules and this is the right thing."

6. Make a list of defiant behaviors on the sheet for the Roadway Book. Select one behavior as the target behavior for the plan.

7. Go over time-out technique.

8. Make goal easily achievable.

9. Select very clear (i.e., specific) rewards.

10. Write out the plan for them to take home and post on the refrigerator.

SNACK

PARENT

1. Talk about reluctance to come to session—see Therapist Form 1: Reluctance Checklist—and ask what tricks the caregiver successfully used to overcome these feelings.

2. Remind her that reluctance is short term and will get better.

3. Ask her to rate her child's reluctance, if any.

HOMEWORK

1. Follow new discipline plan.

2. Mother's homework might be to catch herself feeling guilty and try to ignore it.

PREVIEW THE NEXT SESSION

Next week you will review the discipline plan and start learning new tools to make the scary feelings/PTSD go away (will work individually next time).

PARENT AND CHILD

1. Welcome child and offer candy.
2. Review discipline plan together in <5 minutes, then split up.

CHILD

1. With child alone, review last session.
2. Link talking about feelings doing the drawing to help decrease scary feelings.
3. Talk about nontraumatic but still scary situation first and ask how child would feel (e.g., go to the park, spend the night at relative's house, go to the doctor).
4. Tape a large sheet to the wall, trace the child's body, and encourage child to draw feelings on it. Write in or draw where feelings are felt. Start with nontrauma situations and then work up to reminders of the trauma (e.g., "Where is it that you feel nervous . . . happy . . . sad . . . mad . . . guilty . . . jealous?").
5. Pull out the Roadway Book sheet and recreate the drawing of feelings on the outline.
6. Tell child that next week they will learn more about feelings and a tool to help with reminders.

SNACK

PARENT

1. Review last session.
2. Review discipline plan in more detail. If not followed, find out why and vigorously address the issues of noncompliance. Establish next plan (same or new).
3. Review feelings that were covered with child. Was any of this information a surprise or new? Were any of the feelings that the child revealed new to the mom?
4. Inquire about mother's feelings related to the trauma.
5. Ask mother to rate reluctance on scale of 1–10.
6. Ask mother what "tricks" she used to overcome her reluctance.
7. Remind mother that reluctance will continue and may get worse, but with time will be better.
8. Explain homework and give homework sheet.

HOMEWORK

Give mother homework check sheet.

PREVIEW THE NEXT SESSION

Child will learn more about feelings and get one more tool to help with reminders.

PARENT AND CHILD

1. Welcome and offer candy.
2. Review discipline plan together in <5 minutes. If completed, praise and put in book. If not, problem-solve how future homework can be facilitated. Then split up.

CHILD

1. Review last session with child on how to identify feelings, including gradations.
2. Teach relaxation exercises; explain first that you will be teaching a relaxation method to help with reminders of the trauma and then you will both practice it.
   • Start with imagery of "happy place"; draw it.
   • Next teach the breathing exercise.
   • Teach the muscle exercise.
   • Perhaps do all together: (1) imagery, (2) slow breathing (including holding breath), and (3) muscle relaxation.
   • Use videotaping to reinforce the relaxation techniques.
3. Explain that the homework is to practice the relaxation technique one time. Sticker reward.
4. Teach scary feelings score and help child fill it out.
5. Homework: Pick one time during the week when they get upset by something, rate it on the scary feelings score, and then practice a relaxation technique.
6. Explain that next week you will work more in the Roadway Book and learn some new things about how to control reactions to reminders.

SNACK

PARENT

1. "What did you notice?"
2. Ask mother if she understood the relaxation techniques. Review the techniques.
3. Inquire whether the memories or feelings that the child revealed were new to her. Ask her if any of the conversation with her child surprised her.
4. Teach her about the child's scary feelings score.
5. Ask her to practice this at home once next week so that they both understand how to use it.
6. During conversation, listen for any distorted thoughts and feelings that the mother may reveal.
7. Revisit mother's reluctance and complete Therapist Form 1: Reluctance Checklist. Inquire about tricks used this time or in the past to overcome the reluctance. Remind mother that reluctance may continue or get worse (for both mother and child). This is short term and will get better.

HOMEWORK

Discipline, relaxation, and thermometer homework with sticker rewards.

PREVIEW THE NEXT SESSION

Will start talking more about child's actual symptoms and how to use the tools he or she has learned.

PARENT AND CHILD

1. Welcome and candy.

2. Review in <5 minutes, then split up.

CHILD

1. Briefly review last session:
   - Discipline.
   - Scary feelings score.
   - Relaxation exercises and practice.

2. Tell the story. Explain that you are going to do something together; need complete story about "what happened." Child needs to help you put the story together to include any missing details. Get baseline reading of scary feelings score.

3. During the telling of the story, ask child how they feel in the moment and in the event: scared, helpless, angry?
   - What happened right before the trauma?
   - Who was there, including pets?
   - Where was everybody and what were they doing?
   - What were first signs of danger? What was child's reaction?
   - Is there anything the child wished they would have done but didn't?
   - Smells, tastes, sounds, sights, textures?

4. After recounting the story, have child rate their anxiety using the scary feelings score. Practice relaxation regardless of score. Create a tentative stimulus hierarchy list of the most distressing moments. Get three to five scary moments.

5. Congratulate child for bravery and a job well done.

6. Place sheets in the Roadway Book.

7. Explain next scary feelings homework; practice relaxation.

SNACK

PARENT

1. "What do you think about what you just saw/heard?"

2. Are mother's feelings of distress evident to child?

3. Do distressful reminders from past traumas happen on a regular basis?

4. Review homework; make sure mother understands the techniques and purpose of the relaxation exercises. If there is already a distressful situation, use that; if not, create a situation. Send mother home with the homework check sheet.

SESSION 6

PARENT AND CHILD

1. Welcome and offer candy.

2. Review together in <5 minutes, then split up.

CHILD

1. Review the importance of last session and praise child for how brave he or she was for telling the whole story. Let child know this will help make scary feelings go away. (If necessary, can go over story to finish getting details.) Explain that we will select an easy memory from the list and remember it until it is no longer scary; the feeling will go away. Get baseline scary feelings score.

2. Have child pick an easy memory from the list and draw a picture of it (use sheet from the Roadway Book). Tell child to stay in the memory of the scene until they are not scared at all.

3. Ask child every 3 minutes or so to rate scary feelings.

4. Use relaxation techniques to help child stay with the scene until the scary feelings go away.

5. After the drawing, ask child to close his or her eyes and imagine being in the situation. (Try it even though may be too hard.) Ask for another scary feelings score; when 2 or 3, can stop exposure. If child stops before then or exposure occurs for more than 5 minutes with no change, reassure child that this takes practice and they will get better at it.

6. Put drawing in book.

7. Safety plan: Learn how to avoid trouble in the future and to know to tell when danger is coming before it happens. The ideal elements of a safety plan are to remove oneself from danger and call for help.

8. Explain exposure homework to child.

9. Preview next session with child; they will move up on the stimulus hierarchy and practice a little harder imaginal exposure.

SNACK

PARENT

1. "What were your thoughts while watching today's session?"

2. Look over last week's homework again; make sure she understands proper use of relaxation techniques. Check if she is still using discipline plan.

3. Review the safety plan with her, as you did with her child.

SESSION 7

PARENT AND CHILD

1. Welcome and offer candy.
2. Ask about practicing real-life exposure, using scary feelings score, and practicing relaxation techniques. In <5 minutes, go over what they did.

CHILD

1. Review old homework again with child.
2. Explain we are going to continue to make scary feelings go away. If child had trouble with the item from last week, repeat it. If not, move up to a harder item on the stimulus hierarchy. Ask for scary feelings score. Then ask child to draw a picture of the medium item on the Roadway worksheet.
3. Tell child to stay in the situation until they are not scared at all. Child can use the relaxation technique to help them stay with the scene until the scary feelings go away.
4. After the drawing is complete, ask child to close his or her eyes and imagine being in the situation.
5. Ask for scary feelings scores at the beginning and at the end. If child stops too soon, or if exposure occurs with no change, reassure child that this is practice and they will get better at it.
6. Place the drawing in the Roadway Book.
7. Review the safety plan from last week. Remind child of danger signals and child's response. Puppets: One puppet is the angry person, the second puppet is the child. Provide a running commentary on the action to emphasize the danger signals. Have the child puppet recognize the danger signals and then enact the safety plan.
8. Next, use only the angry puppet as child role-plays the child's part. Display the danger signals and ask child to identify them. Ask the child puppet what they will do for the safety plan.
9. Preview: Let child know that next week he or she will move up a bit on the scary feelings score and practice a little harder imaginal exposure.

PARENT

If it has become apparent that the mother seems preoccupied by her own past experiences, to the detriment of maximizing her resources to focus on her child, consider addressing it. Think about it aloud with the mother: that mothers might need to process their own pasts before they can devote maximal resources to their traumatized child. Listen only; draw no conclusions, other than the need to pay attention to this in the future.

1. Ask mother her thoughts after watching the child's session.
2. Address safety planning for both her child and herself.
3. Discuss old homework; make sure parent still understands purpose of relaxation exercises.
4. If there was a new discipline plan, review it.
5. Rate mother's reluctance; what tricks did she use to overcome it? Remind her that reluctance will continue and may get worse.
6. Explain new homework to mother and child together and give homework check sheet.

PARENT AND CHILD

1. Offer candy and then put it away, as usual.

2. Ask how the homework went in <5 minutes. Did child practice the real-life exposure?

CHILD

1. Review again how the homework was for child in case he or she wants to say anything in private.

2. Explain that together, you are going to continue to make the scary feelings go away. If child had trouble with the item from last week, repeat it. If not, move up to a harder item on the stimulus hierarchy (Child Worksheet 5.2: The Stimulus Hierarchy).

3. Ask child to draw a picture of the medium item on Child Worksheet 5.2. Tell child to stay in the situation until he or she is not scared at all. Child can use the relaxation technique to help him or her stay with the scene until the scary feelings go away.

4. After the drawing is complete, ask child to close his or her eyes and imagine being in the situation. This may be hard, but try it anyway as a trial.

5. Ask for scary feelings scores at the beginning and end. Practice relaxation. If child stops before the end, or if exposure occurs with no change, reassure child that this is practice and he or she will get better at it.

6. Place the drawing in the Roadway Book.

7. Review the safety plan. Role-play the danger signals with the puppet again. Have child identify the danger signals and rehearse his or her safety plan.

8. Let child know that next week he or she will move up a bit on the scary feelings score and practice a little harder imaginal exposure.

PARENT

1. Ask mother for her thoughts after watching the child's sessions.

2. Allow mother an open-ended opportunity to talk about what she just heard from her child or to talk about her own feelings and memories.

3. Discuss old homework with her and make sure she still understands the purpose of the relaxation exercises.

4. Discuss the (new) discipline plan and whether child's behavior has improved or not.

5. Ask mother to rate her reluctance (Therapist Form 1: Reluctance Checklist), what tricks she used to overcome it, and remind her that reluctance will continue and may get worse.

6. Explain the homework to mother and child together and give mother the homework check sheet.

SESSION 9

PARENT AND CHILD

1. Welcome both and offer candy to child.

2. Review the homework: disciplining defiant behavior, responding to the medium exposure, rehearsing the safety plan.

CHILD

1. Review the homework. Did child practice the real-life exposure? Discuss in detail.

2. Explain that this will be like last week, to make scary feelings go away. If child had trouble with the item last week, start with that one again. If not, move up to the worst moment.

3. Get the baseline rating.

4. Ask child to draw a picture of almost the worst moment. Tell child to stay with the situation until he or she is not scared. If closing his or her eyes has worked previously, ask child to imagine this moment; if not, ask child to look at his or her picture. Get a rating. Practice the relaxation exercises. Repeat until the rating is low.

5. Explain the homework.

6. Safety planning: Ask child if he or she practiced the safety plan from last week. How did it go? If it was not practiced, why not? Troubleshoot. Review the danger signals and what child can do in response.

7. Tell child that next week, you will all review the Roadway Book together: child, his or her mother, and you.

PARENT

1. "What were your thoughts and feelings after watching the session?"

2. Discuss the old homework. Make sure parent understands the purpose of the relaxation exercises.

3. Address safety planning with parent.

4. Ask mother to rate her reluctance prior to coming to appointment (Therapist Form 1: Reluctance Checklist) and what tricks she used to overcome it.

5. Explain the homework to mother and child and give mother the homework check sheet.

PARENT AND CHILD

1. Welcome parent and child and offer the child candy.

2. How did the homework go? Did the child practice real-life exposure?

CHILD

1. Review the homework with child.

2. Explain that like last week, together you are going to make the scary feelings go away. If child had trouble with the item last week, start with that one again. If not, move up to the worst moment.

3. Get child's baseline rating.

4. Ask child to draw a picture of the worst moment. Tell child to stay with the situation until he or she is no longer scared. If eyes closed worked for child, ask him or her to imagine the moment; if not, ask child to look at his or her drawing. Get child's anxiety rating using the scary feelings score. Have child practice relaxation until the rating is low.

5. Place the drawing in the Roadway Book.

6. Tell child that next week you will talk about planning for the future.

PARENT

1. "What were your thoughts and feelings after watching the session?"

2. Discuss old homework. Make sure next week parent understands purpose of the relaxation exercises.

3. Ask mother for her reluctance rating (Therapist Form 1: Reluctance Checklist) and what tricks she used to overcome the reluctance.

4. Explain the new homework to mother and child together and give the homework check sheet to mother.

PARENT AND CHILD

Review Sessions 1–6 in the Roadway Book. Cover each page carefully; remind child of the purpose and learning reflected on each page. Offer praise for accomplishments. (Should take 5–15 minutes.)

Tell them only two more sessions left. Need to start saying goodbye. Next week, talk more about this and how to use the tools learned in the future.

PARENT AND CHILD

1. Welcome, give candy.

2. Review the last session and how the homework went.

CHILD

1. Remind child that a lot of scary, bad memories have gone away and no longer bother him or her, but that sometimes these memories will pop back up and scare the child.

2. Ask child to think of events in the near future that might make bad memories pop back up. If child cannot think of something, suggest something and tell a story with the example. Have child draw the situation.

3. Ask child what tools he or she would use to cope with it. What would he or she do?

4. Ask child to draw a picture of him- or herself all grown up and to try and think of a situation then that might bring back the scary, bad memories. Have child draw a picture of the situation. Ask how child might handle the situation. What tools would he or she use?

5. Ask child for a scary feelings score.

6. Let child know that next week is graduation; ask about small treat child might like.

PARENT

1. Discuss old homework with parent. Make sure parent still understands the purpose of the relaxation exercises.

2. Remind mother that the next session is the last one; explain that they ought to bring closure to the events they have been talking about over the previous weeks. Offer an open-ended or guided discussion.

3. Ask mother to rate her reluctance (Therapist Form 1: Reluctance Checklist).

4. What tricks does she use to overcome her reluctance?

PARENT AND CHILD

1. Review the rest of the Roadway Book.

2. Explain the homework to mother and child together: another real-life exposure to practice.

   Remind them again that next week is the last session.

(Photocopy the Roadway Book sheets prior to the next session so that you can keep a copy.)

PARENT AND CHILD

1. Have parent fill out the weekly symptoms checklist (Therapist Form 2: Scary Feelings Score Form).

2. Welcome them and offer candy to child.

3. Review the last session and how the last homework went. Encourage child by recounting all that he or she has learned and how child can use the skills in other areas of life.

4. Photocopy the last page of homework.

5. Review the Roadway Book (all sessions). Encourage empowerment and give child the book at the end.

6. Give child a certificate of completion.

7. Offer a small treat.

8. Take a photo of child and you, if appropriate.

9. Ask mother for a final rating of her and her child's reluctance.

References

Achenbach, T. M., & Rescorla, L. A. (2000). *Manual for the ASEBA preschool forms and profiles.* Burlington: University of Vermont, Research Center for Children, Youth, & Families.

Allen, A., Saltzman, W. R., Brymer, M. J., Oshri, A., & Silverman, W. K. (2006). An empirically informed intervention for children following exposure to severe hurricanes. *The Behavior Therapist, 29*(6), 118–124.

American Psychiatric Association. (1980). *Diagnostic and statistical manual of mental disorders* (3rd ed.). Washington, DC: Author.

American Psychiatric Association. (1987). *Diagnostic and statistical manual of mental disorders* (3rd ed., rev.). Washington, DC: Author.

American Psychiatric Association. (2013). *Diagnostic and statistical manual of mental disorders* (5th ed.). Arlington, VA: Author.

Ancoli, S., & Kamiya, J. (1979). Respiratory patterns during emotional expression. *Biofeedback and Self-Regulation, 4,* 242.

Ancoli, S., Kamiya, J., & Ekman, P. (1980). Psychophysiological differentiation of positive and negative affects. *Biofeedback and Self-Regulation, 5,* 356–357.

Angold, A., Costello, E. J., Farmer, E. M. Z., Burns, B. J., & Erkanli, A. (1999). Impaired but undiagnosed. *Journal of the American Academy of Child and Adolescent Psychiatry, 38*(2), 129–137.

Bandura, A. (1969). *Principles of behavior modification.* New York: Holt, Rinehart & Winston.

Beck, A. T. (1967). *Depression: Clinical, experimental, and theoretical aspects.* New York: Harper & Row.

Bogat, G. A., DeJonghe, E., Levendosky, A. A., Davidson, W. S., & von Eye, A. (2006). Trauma symptoms among infants exposed to intimate partner violence. *Child Abuse and Neglect, 30,* 109–125.

Bonanno, G. A., Mancini, A. D., Horton, J. L., Powell, T. M., Leardmann, C. A., Boyko, E. J., et al. (2012). Trajectories of trauma symptoms and resilience in deployed U.S. military service members: Prospective cohort study. *British Journal of Psychiatry, 200*(4), 317–323.

Briere, J. (2005). *Trauma Symptom Checklist for Young Children (TSCYC): Professional manual.* Lutz, FL: Psychological Assessment Resources.

Briere, J., Johnson, K., Bissada, A., Damon, L., Crouch, J., Gil, E., et al. (2001). The Trauma Symptom Checklist for Young Children (TSCYC): Reliability and association with abuse exposure in a multi-site study. *Child Abuse and Neglect, 25*(8), 1001–1014.

Carrion, V. G., Weems, C. F., Ray, R., & Reiss, A. L. (2002). Toward an empirical definition of pediatric PTSD:

The phenomenology of PTSD symptoms in youth. *Journal of the American Academy of Child and Adolescent Psychiatry, 41*(2), 166–173.

CATS Consortium. (2007). Implementing CBT for traumatized children and adolescents after September 11: Lessons learned from the Child and Adolescent Trauma Treatment Services (CATS) project. *Journal of Clinical Child and Adolescent Psychology, 36*(4), 581–592.

Cloitre, M., Stolbach, B. C., Herman, J. L., van der Kolk, B. A., Pynoos, R. S., Wang, J., et al. (2009). A developmental approach to complex PTSD: Childhood and adult cumulative trauma as predictors of symptom complexity. *Journal of Traumatic Stress, 22*(5), 399–408.

Cohen, J. A., & the American Academy of Child and Adolescent Psychiatry, Work Group on Quality Issues. (1998). Practice parameters for the assessment and treatment of children and adolescents with posttraumatic stress disorder. *Journal of the American Academy of Child and Adolescent Psychiatry, 37*(10, Suppl.), 4S–26S.

Cohen, J. A., & Mannarino, A. P. (1996a). A treatment outcome study for sexually abused preschool children: Initial findings. *Journal of the American Academy of Child and Adolescent Psychiatry, 35*, 42–50.

Cohen, J. A., & Mannarino, A. P. (1996b). Factors that mediate treatment outcome of sexually abused preschool children. *Journal of the American Academy of Child and Adolescent Psychiatry, 34*, 1402–1410.

Cohen, J. A., & Scheeringa, M. S. (2009). Post-traumatic stress disorder diagnosis in children: Challenges and promises. *Dialogues in Clinical Neuroscience, 11*(1), 91–99.

Copeland, W. E., Keeler, G., Angold, A., & Costello, E. J. (2007). Traumatic events and posttraumatic stress in childhood. *Archives of General Psychiatry, 64*, 577–584.

Deblinger, E., Stauffer, L. B., & Steer, R. A. (2001). Comparative efficacies of supportive and cognitive behavioral group therapies for young children who have been sexually abused and their nonoffending mothers. *Child Maltreatment, 6*, 332–343.

Dehon, C., & Scheeringa, M. S. (2006). Screening for preschool posttraumatic stress disorder with the Child Behavior Checklist. *Journal of Pediatric Psychology, 31*(4), 431–435.

DeVoe, E. R., Bannon, W. M., Jr., & Klein, T. P. (2006). Post-9/11 helpseeking by New York City parents on behalf of highly exposed young children. *American Journal of Orthopsychiatry, 76*(2), 167–175.

De Young, A. C., Drury, S. S., Scheeringa, M. S. (in press). Assessing trauma-related symptoms during early childhood. In R. DelCarmen-Wiggins & A. Carter (Eds.), *Handbook of infant, toddler, and preschool mental health assessment* (2nd ed.) New York: Oxford University Press.

De Young, A. C., Kenardy, J. A., Cobham, V. E., & Kimble, R. (2012). Prevalence, comorbidity and course of trauma reactions in young burn-injured children. *Journal of Child Psychology and Psychiatry, 53*(1), 56–63.

Egger, H. L., Erkanli, A., Keeler, G., Potts, E., Walter, B. K., & Angold, A. (2006). Test–retest reliability of the Preschool Age Psychiatric Assessment (PAPA). *Journal of the American Academy of Child and Adolescent Psychiatry, 45*(5), 538–549.

Fauerbauch, J. A., Lawrence, J. W., Schmidt, C. W., Munster, A. M., & Costa, P. T. (2000). Personality predictors of injury-related posttraumatic stress disorder. *Journal of Nervous and Mental Disease, 188*, 510–517.

Feldman, R., & Vengrober, A. (2011). Posttraumatic stress disorder in infants and young children exposed to war-related trauma. *Journal of the American Academy of Child and Adolescent Psychiatry, 50*(7), 645–658.

Finkelhor, D., Ormrod, R. K., & Turner, H. A. (2007). Poly-victimization: A neglected component in child victimization. *Child Abuse and Neglect, 31*(1), 7–26.

Finkelhor, D., Vanderminden, J., Turner, H., Hamby, S., & Shattuck, A. (2014). Upset among youth in response to questions about exposure to violence, sexual assault, and family maltreatment. *Child Abuse and Neglect, 38*(2), 217–223.

Fivush, R. (1993). Developmental perspectives on autobiographical recall. In G. Goodman & B. Bottoms (Eds.), *Child victims, child witnesses: Understanding and improving testimony* (pp. 1–24). New York: Guilford Press.

Foa, E. B., Keane, T. M., Friedman, M. J., & Cohen, J. A. (2009). *Effective treatments for PTSD: Practice guidelines from the International Society for Traumatic Stress Studies* (2nd ed.). New York: Guilford Press.

Ford, J. D., Connor, D. F., & Hawke, J. (2009). Complex trauma among psychiatrically impaired children: A cross-sectional, chart-review study. *Journal of Clinical Psychiatry, 70*(8), 1155–1163.

Ghosh-Ippen, C. G., Briscoe-Smith, A., & Lieberman, A. F. (2004, November). *PTSD symptomatology in young children.* Paper presented at the 20th annual meeting of the International Society for Traumatic Stress Studies, New Orleans, LA.

Graf, A., Schiestl, C., & Landolt, M. A. (2011). Posttraumatic stress and behavior problems in infants and toddlers with burns. *Journal of Pediatric Psychology, 36*(8), 923–931.

Grave, J., & Blissett, J. (2004). Is cognitive behavior therapy developmentally appropriate for young children?: A critical review of the evidence. *Clinical Psychology Review, 24*, 399–420.

Gross, J., & Hayne, H. (1998). Drawing facilitates children's verbal reports of emotionally laden events. *Journal of Experimental Psychology, 4*, 163–179.

Hickman, L. J., Jaycox, L. H., Setodji, C. M., Kofner, A., Schultz, D., Barnes-Proby, D., et al. (2012). How much does "how much" matter?: Assessing the relationship between children's lifetime exposure to violence and trauma symptoms, behavior problems, and parenting stress. *Journal of Interpersonal Violence, 28*(6), 1338–1362.

Hodges, M., Godbout, N., Briere, J., Lanktree, C., Gilbert, A., & Kletzka, N. T. (2013). Cumulative trauma and symptom complexity in children: A path analysis. *Child Abuse and Neglect, 37*, 891–898.

Kilpatrick, K. L., & Resnick, H. S. (1993). Posttraumatic stress disorder associated with exposure to criminal victimization in clinical and community populations. In J. Davidson & E. Foa (Eds.), *Posttraumatic stress disorder: DSM-IV and beyond* (pp. 113–143). Washington, DC: American Psychiatric Association.

Kollins, S., Greenhill, L. L., Swanson, J. M., Wigal, S., Abikoff, H. B., McCracken, J., et al. (2006). Rationale, design, and methods of the Preschool ADHD Treatment Study (PATS). *Journal of the American Academy of Child and Adolescent Psychiatry, 45*(11), 1275–1283.

Levendosky, A. A., Huth-Bocks, A. C., Semel, M. A., & Shapiro, D. L. (2002). Trauma symptoms in preschool-age children exposed to domestic violence. *Journal of Interpersonal Violence, 17*(2), 150–164.

MacLean, G. (1977). Psychic trauma and traumatic neurosis: Play therapy with a four-year-old boy. *Canadian Psychiatric Association Journal, 22*, 71–75.

MacLean, G. (1980). Addendum to a case of traumatic neurosis: Consideration of family dynamics. *Canadian Journal of Psychiatry, 25*, 506–508.

Malchiodi, C. A. (1997). *Breaking the silence: Art therapy with children from violent homes.* New York: Brunner/Mazel.

March, J. S., Amaya-Jackson, L., Murray, M. C., & Schulte, A. (1998). Cognitive-behavioral psychotherapy for children and adolescents with posttraumatic stress disorder after a single-incident stressor. *Journal of the American Academy of Child and Adolescent Psychiatry, 37*, 585–593.

McFarlane, A. C. (1989). The aetiology of post-traumatic morbidity: Predisposing, precipitating and perpetuating factors. *British Journal of Psychiatry, 154*, 221–228.

Measelle, J. R., Ablow, J. C., Cowan, P. A., & Cowan, C. P. (1998). Assessing young children's views of their academic, social, and emotional lives: An evaluation of the self-perception scales of the Berkeley Puppet Interview. *Child Development, 69*(6), 1556–1576.

Meiser-Stedman, R., Smith, P., Glucksman, E., Yule, W., & Dalgleish, T. (2008). The posttraumatic stress disorder diagnosis in preschool- and elementary school-age children exposed to motor vehicle accidents. *American Journal of Psychiatry, 165*(10), 1326–1337.

National Institute for Clinical Excellence. (2005). *Post-traumatic stress disorder: The management of PTSD in adults and children in primary and secondary care.* London: Author.

Neugebauer, R., Wasserman, G. A., Fisher, P. W., Kline, J., Geller, P. A., & Miller, L. S. (1999). Darryl, a cartoon-based measure of cardinal posttraumatic stress symptoms in school-age children. *American Journal of Public Health, 89*, 758–761.

Nilsson, D. K., Gustafsson, P. E., & Svedin, C. G. (2012). Polytraumatization and trauma symptoms in adolescent boys and girls: Interpersonal and noninterpersonal events and moderating effects of adverse family circumstances. *Journal of Interpersonal Violence, 27*(13), 2645–2664.

References

Ohmi, H., Kojima, S., Awai, Y., Kamata, S., Sasaki, K., Tanaka, Y., et al. (2002). Post-traumatic stress disorder in pre-school aged children after a gas explosion. *European Journal of Pediatrics, 161*(12), 643–648.

Pollio, E. S., Glover-Orr, L. E., & Wherry, J. N. (2008). Assessing posttraumatic stress disorder using the Trauma Symptom Checklist for Young Children. *Journal of Child Sexual Abuse, 17*(1), 89–100.

Pruett, K. D. (1979). Home treatment for two infants who witnessed their mother's murder. *Journal of the American Academy of Child Psychiatry, 18*, 647–657.

Rimm, D. C., & Masters, I. C. (1979). *Behavior therapy: Techniques and empirical findings.* Orlando, FL: Academic Press.

Roth, S., Newman, E., Pelcovitz, D., van der Kolk, B. A., & Mandel, F. S. (1997). Complex PTSD in victims exposed to sexual and physical abuse: Results from the DSM-IV field trial for posttraumatic stress disorder. *Journal of Traumatic Stress, 10*(4), 539–555.

Rothbaum, B. O., & Foa, E. B. (1996). Cognitive-behavioral therapy for posttraumatic stress disorder. In B. A. van der Kolk, A. C. McFarlane, & L. Weisaeth (Eds.), *Traumatic stress: The effects of overwhelming experience on mind, body, and society* (pp. 491–509). New York: Guilford Press.

Runyon, M. K., Basilio, I., Van Hasselt, V. B., & Hersen, M. (1998). Child witnesses of interparental violence: Child and family treatment. In V. B. Van Hasselt & M. Hersen (Eds.), *Handbook of psychological treatment protocols for children and adolescents* (pp. 203–278). Mahwah, NJ: Erlbaum.

Salloum, A. (1998). *Reactions: A workbook to help young people who are experiencing trauma and grief.* Omaha, NE: Centering Corporation.

Scheeringa, M. S. (2010). *Young Child PTSD Checklist.* New Orleans: Tulane University School of Medicine.

Scheeringa, M. S. (2011). PTSD in children younger than age of 13: Towards a developmentally sensitive diagnosis. *Journal of Child and Adolescent Trauma, 4*(3), 181–197.

Scheeringa, M. S. (2015). Untangling psychiatric comorbidity in young children who experienced single, repeated, or Hurricane Katrina traumatic events. *Child and Youth Care Forum, 44*(4), 475–492.

Scheeringa, M. S., & Haslett, N. (2010). The reliability and criterion validity of the Diagnostic Infant and Preschool Assessment: A new diagnostic instrument for young children. *Child Psychiatry and Human Development, 41*(3), 299–312.

Scheeringa, M. S., Myers, L., Putnam, F. W., & Zeanah, C. H. (2012). Diagnosing PTSD in early childhood: An empirical assessment of four approaches. *Journal of Traumatic Stress, 25*(4), 359–367.

Scheeringa, M. S., Myers, L., Putnam, F. W., & Zeanah, C. H. (2015). Maternal factors as moderators or mediators of PTSD symptoms in preschool children: A two-year prospective study. *Journal of Family Violence, 30*(5), 633–642.

Scheeringa, M. S., Peebles, C. D., Cook, C. A., & Zeanah, C. H. (2001). Toward establishing procedural, criterion, and discriminant validity for PTSD in early childhood. *Journal of the American Academy of Child and Adolescent Psychiatry, 40*(1), 52–60.

Scheeringa, M. S., Salloum, A., Arnberger, R. A., Weems, C. F., Amaya-Jackson, L., & Cohen, J. A. (2007). Feasibility and effectiveness of cognitive-behavioral therapy for posttraumatic stress disorder in preschool children: Two case reports. *Journal of Traumatic Stress, 20*(4), 631–636.

Scheeringa, M. S., Weems, C. F., Cohen, J. A., Amaya-Jackson, L., & Guthrie, D. (2011). Trauma-focused cognitive-behavioral therapy for posttraumatic stress disorder in three through six year-old children: A randomized clinical trial. *Journal of Child Psychology and Psychiatry, 52*(8), 853–860.

Scheeringa, M. S., Wright, M. J., Hunt, J. P., & Zeanah, C. H. (2006). Factors affecting the diagnosis and prediction of PTSD symptomatology in children and adolescents. *American Journal of Psychiatry, 163*(4), 644–651.

Scheeringa, M. S., & Zeanah, C. H. (2001). A relational perspective on PTSD in early childhood. *Journal of Traumatic Stress, 14*, 799–815.

Scheeringa, M. S., & Zeanah, C. H. (2008). Reconsideration of harm's way: Onsets and comorbidy patterns of disorders in preschool children and their caregivers following Hurricane Katrina. *Journal of Clinical Child and Adolescent Psychology, 37*(3), 508–518.

Scheeringa, M. S., Zeanah, C. H., & Cohen, J. A. (2011). PTSD in children and adolescents: Toward an empirically based algorithm. *Depression and Anxiety, 28*(9), 770–782.

Scheeringa, M. S., Zeanah, C. H., Drell, M. J., & Larrieu, J. A. (1995). Two approaches to the diagnosis of post-traumatic stress disorder in infancy and early childhood. *Journal of the American Academy of Child and Adolescent Psychiatry, 34*, 191–200.

Scheeringa, M. S., Zeanah, C. H., Myers, L., & Putnam, F. W. (2003). New findings on alternative criteria for PTSD in preschool children. *Journal of the American Academy of Child and Adolescent Psychiatry, 42*(5), 561–570.

Scheeringa, M. S., Zeanah, C. H., Myers, L., & Putnam, F. W. (2005). Predictive validity in a prospective follow-up of PTSD in preschool children. *Journal of the American Academy of Child and Adolescent Psychiatry, 44*(9), 899–906.

Silverman, W. K., Ortiz, C. D., Viswesvaran, C., Burns, B. J., Kolko, D. J., Putnam, F. W., et al. (2008). Evidence-based psychosocial treatments for children and adolescents exposed to traumatic events. *Journal of Clinical Child and Adolescent Psychology, 37*(1), 156–183.

Skinner, B. F. (1953). *Science and human behavior.* New York: Free Press.

Steele, W. (2012). Using drawing in short-term trauma resolution. In C. A. Malchiodi (Ed.), *Handbook of art therapy* (2nd ed., pp. 162–174). New York: Guilford Press.

Stoddard, F. J., Saxe, G., Ronfeldt, H., Drake, J. E., Burns, J., Edgren, C., et al. (2006). Acute stress symptoms in young children with burns. *Journal of the American Academy of Child and Adolescent Psychiatry, 45*(1), 87–93.

Terr, L. C. (1988). What happens to early memories of trauma?: A study of twenty children under age five at the time of documented traumatic events. *Journal of the American Academy of Child and Adolescent Psychiatry, 27*(1), 96–104.

Thase, M. E., & Wright, J. H. (1997). Cognitive and behavioral therapies. In A. Tasman, J. Kay, & J. A. Lieberman (Eds.), *Psychiatry* (pp. 1418–1438). Philadelphia: Saunders.

van der Kolk, B. A. (2005). Developmental trauma disorder. *Psychiatric Annals, 35*(5), 401–408.

Weems, C. F., Costa, N. M., & Watts, S. E. (2007). Cognitive errors, anxiety sensitivity, and anxiety control beliefs: Their unique and specific associations with childhood anxiety symptoms. *Behavior Modification, 31*(2), 174–201.

Weems, C. F., & Scheeringa, M. S. (2013). Maternal depression and treatment gains following a cognitive behavioral intervention for posttraumatic stress in preschool children. *Journal of Anxiety Disorders, 27*(1), 140–146.

Wolfe, V. V., Gentile, C., & Wolfe, D. A. (1989). The impact of sexual abuse on children: A PTSD formulation. *Behavior Therapy, 20*(2), 215–228.

Zoellner, L. A., Fitzgibbons, L. A., & Foa, E. B. (2001). Cognitive-behavioral approaches to PTSD. In J. P. Wilson, M. J. Friedman, & J. D. Lindy (Eds.), *Treating psychological trauma and PTSD* (pp. 159–182). New York: Guilford Press.

Index

Note: *t* following a page number indicates a table.